Finding the Way

Antibiotic Overload, Chemicals and Toxins, and Processed Foods are Collectively Destroying the Health of Our Children. Learn the Facts and Transform Your Child's Health for a Lifetime.

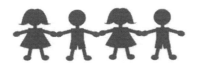

Elizabeth DeRosa

ISBN: 149477111X
ISBN 13: 9781494771119
Library of Congress Control Number: 2015903155
CreateSpace Independent Publishing Platform
North Charleston, South Carolina

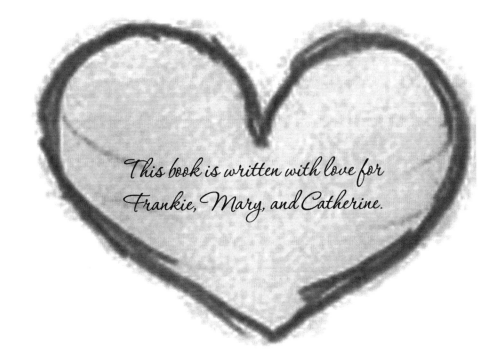

This book is written with love for
Frankie, Mary, and Catherine.

Table of Contents

Acknowledgments:

I want to give a huge thank you to my brother, Jamie Clifford, for his time, ideas, suggestions, and critiques on this project. He walked me through the process of writing and how to navigate my way through the publishing world. I would be remiss if I did not point out that Jamie is the storyteller in our family. His fictional works can be found at www.jrclifford.com.

Thank you to Jitka Terhaerdt (www.jitkaphoto.zenfolio.com) and Jen Reilly for taking some of the pictures included in this book.

Thank you to the Great Pumpkin Market for generously allowing me to use their products in some of the photographs throughout this book.

Frank, you are and always will be the love of my life. Thank you for having the courage to allow me to share some of our family's personal stories with the world.

Dr. B, thank you for your guidance and knowledge into the world of holistic health. You have given Frankie an opportunity to live his life without physical limitations. I will be forever grateful!

Mary and Catherine, thank you for showing me the world through the lens of a child again. You are both colorful gifts.

Frankie, you are a hero to me. To overcome the physical limitations that ten years of illness brought you at such a young age is a testament to your inner courage and strength. Both of these qualities are immeasurable and truly personify your soaring spirit. I hope you carry these gifts with you to share with the world. You are my teacher! ILY

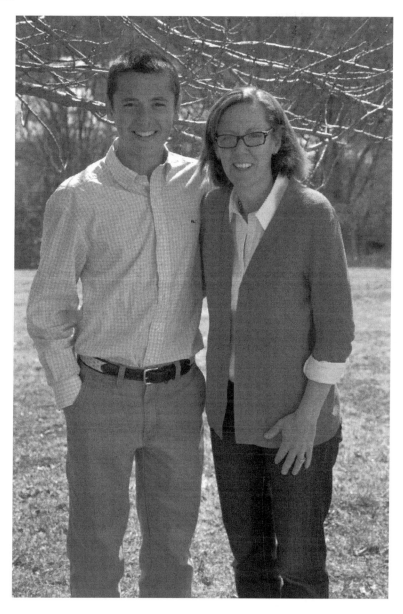

Introduction:

"While we try to teach our children all about life, our children teach us what life is all about."
—ANGELA SCHWINDT

Mahatma Gandhi once said, "Be the change you want to see in this world." To many people the word change can often be associated with scary and overwhelming thoughts, fears, and feelings. To change the way one views the world means one might have to look at something from a different perspective or point of view. Allowing yourself the opportunity to look at something from a different point of view, both externally and internally, suggests you are open to the possibility of change. Whether we like it or not, change is a part of life. I have come to engage and accept change in a powerful, life-altering way. I thought change entered my life in a dramatic, somewhat unwelcome way. However, by slowly embracing this change, my life and my family's life has profoundly shifted and evolved.

By changing the medical treatment plan for my son, a whole new holistic world has opened up to us. I have chosen to share our story because I feel deeply passionate about the message it conveys.

This book focuses on five key points:

1. The prevalence of health issues facing children today.
2. The connection to health from the chemical and toxic barrage our children face in their daily environment.
3. Ideas on ways to eliminate this chemical barrage including looking at healthy choices in food, water, beauty supplies, and cleaning products.
4. Basic insights into nutrition, your body, and the importance of a healthy digestive system. This includes issues of Candida (inner body yeast infection) and antibiotic overload.
5. Practical solutions, suggestions, and resources to assist you (This is my attempt to introduce the importance of incorporating and understanding holistic health approaches as an alternative to the "mainstream" way of controlling and fighting disease).

In deciding to write this book I contemplated, prayed over, and questioned what my main purpose would be. I asked myself, "Why would I want to take the time to write and research a book about the topics we will explore? How can I write such a book when I am not an expert on any of the issues I will present to you?" I often wonder how many other families are out there searching for clues about their child's health with limited answers provided by their pediatrician or medical specialist. How many parents actually comprehend what their children are eating on a daily basis and how what they eat can have long lasting negative effects on their health? What is the connection between our children's daily environment and their overall health? How can I share our story in a way that encourages other families to seek the answers they need regarding their child's overall well-being?

The simple answer to all of these questions is that this book exists because I have lived it with my son and family. Together, we have experienced over ten years of chronic, physical symptoms that disappeared after the introduction of a more holistic or natural approach to health. At the age of forty-four, I have discovered one of my life's purposes: to bring awareness and information to individuals and families about the dangers of the overuse and continuous use of antibiotics and medications, the existing problems with the country's food supply, the importance of clean and nutritious food, and what we can do to limit our children's exposure to toxic chemicals in their daily environment. It is my genuine and heartfelt belief that if the information found in this book can assist one child or family who is suffering needlessly with chronic and daily physical symptoms then it has absolutely—without question—served its purpose. I did not begin this writing project with the intent to share it and its content with others. As I began educating myself on the issues discussed in this book, I felt an overwhelming desire to follow my heart and make it available to all.

This medical journey with my son has been life altering and uplifting for me in many different, yet profoundly important ways. This book started out as a journal I will one day share with Frankie as gets older and becomes more independent from me. He may not always want to hear what "Mom" has to say, but he can always read or look through this writing project with an open heart and mind if he so chooses. My daughters, Mary and Catherine, now too have been given some basic insight into and tools for living a healthier life. I have begun to shift my family's understanding of the environment (physical, emotional, and spiritual). It is my hope they carry and reflect on some of these ideas as they grow and mature.

Your child does not need to present with daily physical symptoms for you to decide that reducing chemicals in his or her daily environment is something that you would like to explore further. Your "healthy" child could benefit as well.

It is my hope that by telling part of our story you gain the knowledge and understanding that our children are facing many challenges in today's world and you can help make a dramatic difference. I invite you to look at the topics discussed in this book and reach out for your own unique answers.

You cannot depend on the food industry, the government, the pharmaceutical industry, or the medical profession to adequately and thoroughly inform you of these very important topics. I may touch on a topic that peaks your curiosity or that you want to explore further. Please know there are other resources available to you that are much more in-depth. Entire books have been dedicated to the topics I talk about briefly in this book.

There are no rules, no boundaries, no right or wrong ways, and no judgment on making some changes in your family's daily environment. Any change you make, large or small, is a step in the right direction. A fundamental belief that change is possible is the stepping stone that unknowingly began this journey for my family.

It is important to understand that I will present you with ideas and limited research to back up a specific school of thought on some important issues. Both sides of the argument claim to have scientific data, charts, statistics, graphs, and the moral high ground on their side. There is always more than one way to look at a situation or issue. It is our job to get the facts, listen to the issues, and make an informed decision on behalf of our children. The problem, as I have witnessed and experienced firsthand, is that most of the time we are only getting information from one side. To be honest, I did not even know there was another side. It is my hope this book lays out a beginning framework for the other side of the argument—the holistic approach to medical care and taking care of ourselves. The majority of this book will focus on one aspect of the holistic approach to medical treatment: the body. I have, however, included a chapter at the end of this book that details my own personal medical crisis and my connection to the entire holistic approach to my diagnosis, surgery, and recovery. This holistic approach encompasses physical, emotional, and spiritual wellness. I included this chapter because I feel strongly that there is a message in my experience as well. I believe my on-going healing journey helps make the connection to the positive benefits of eating the right foods and taking care of ourselves. If you wish to not deviate from the main theme of this book and read just about the physical approach to holistic care, I suggest skipping Chapter 15 when you get there and moving straight to chapter 16.

I have included a list of resources for you in some of the chapters as well as in the back of this book. I have expanded the resource list with you in mind. I feel it is important to provide a wide range of options for you to consider and explore. There are thousands upon thousands of resources out there for you. I have only begun to scratch the surface.

I have utilized many resources to help me better understand and implement the changes we as a family have made together. Documentaries, the Internet, books, and talking with professionals in the field of nutrition and health were my main tools in gathering information. If you feel that there is something missing from this book—and believe me, there is—I encourage you to search further for yourself. This book is being offered to you only as a starting point.

The information in this book does not and should not act as a medical reference for you or your child. Please seek professional guidance in regard to your physical health and well-being. I am not a medical expert. I can tell you though that our physical bodies are all uniquely different and require specific medical and nutritional plans to sustain maximum health. I do not have all of the answers for my family, let alone your families. This book has not been written to tell you how to live. It has not been written to tell you I am doing it right and you are doing it wrong. The last five years has been a personal journey that has seen significant challenges, changes, power struggles, tantrums (parent and child), and frustrations.

The changes that have taken place in my family have been challenging to say the least. I wrote this book because I am a concerned mother who is beginning to make the connection between our children's health, our health, and the often toxic environment we are living in today and that we will pass on to our children and future generations.

I believe one of the greatest gifts I can pass on to my children is an awareness of the importance of healthy eating and of what they are eating.

I wish you continued Blessings to you and yours. May abundant and vibrant health be with you always!

Love,
Elizabeth

I have left a few pages blank for your personal use as you navigate your way through this book. It is my hope you will use these pages to write down your thoughts, questions, and ideas that may need more of your personal attention or continued research for you or your child.

NOTES:

NOTES:

Take a few minutes and write down some ideas or thoughts on what changes you would like to make for your child and family. Please feel free to come back to this list to add anything that resonates with you.

_____

_____

_____

_____

_____

_____

_____

_____

_____

_____

Take a few minutes and think about some of the health issues you or your child is struggling with now or in the past. These health issues can be physical, emotional, or behavioral in nature. Write them down and include as many symptoms as you can recall. List what you are doing or have done in the past to treat symptoms.

Example:

Diagnosis: Environmental allergies. He was diagnosed at age 3.

Symptoms: Congestion, cough, watery eyes, dark circles under eyes, and sneezing.

Duration of Symptoms: On-going and sporadic.

Medications/antibiotics: Claritin, Zyrtec, Singulair, nasal sprays, Amoxicillin, Zithromax, Orapred, and Augmentin.

Other types of treatment: Saline nasal rinses, Mucinex, nebulizer machine, humidifiers, air purifiers, allergy-free bedding, air-duct cleaning, Motrin and Advil, and daily food and weather logs.

Procedures: Allergy testing and blood testing completed several times over the years. Negative test results each time. Countless doctor visits, peak-flow meter readings, and chest x-rays.

Doctors: Pediatrician, allergy specialist, and ENT.

Diagnosis: _____

Symptoms: _____

_____

Duration of Symptoms: _____

_____

Medications/Antibiotics: _____

_____

Other Types of Treatment: _____

Doctors: _____

Diagnosis: _____

Symptoms: _____

_____

Duration of Symptoms: _____

_____

Medications/Antibiotics: _____

_____

Other Types of Treatment: _____

Doctors: _____

Diagnosis: _____

Symptoms: _____

_____

Duration of Symptoms: _____

_____

Medications/Antibiotics: _____

_____

Other Types of Treatment: _____

Doctors: _____

Pick one or two days out of your child's or children's schedule and write down everything they eat. Be sure to include drinks, condiments, and snacks. Pick a day that will give you the best picture of what your child is eating on a regular basis.

Date: _____

Breakfast: _____

Snack: _____

Lunch: _____

Snack: _____

Dinner: _____

Snack: _____

Drinks: _____

Date: _____

Breakfast: _____

Snack: _____

Lunch: _____

Snack: _____

Dinner: _____

Snack: _____

Drinks: _____

Date: _____

Breakfast: _____

Snack: _____

Lunch: _____

Snack: _____

Dinner: _____

Snack: _____

Drinks: _____

Date: _____

Breakfast: _____

Snack: _____

Lunch: _____

Snack: _____

Dinner: _____

Snack: _____

Drinks: _____

Section 1
Here We Go

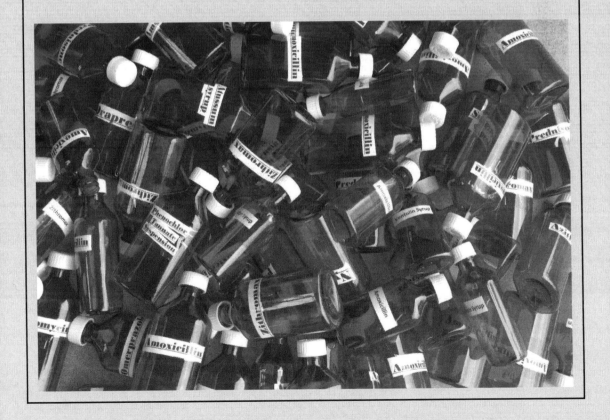

CHAPTER 1
The Starting Point

"Two roads diverged in the woods, and I took the one less traveled by, and that has made all the difference."
—ROBERT FROST

This book reveals my family's journey through my son's medical abyss and the incredible physical healing that transformed his health after being diagnosed with asthma and allergies for years and years. Frankie suffered for over a decade with symptoms, conditions, ailments, and numerous diagnoses. The writing in this book lays out my family's story and the incredible health transformation that occurred by opening ourselves up to change and new ways of doing things. By learning about and integrating holistic health practices into our daily life and letting go of some modern medical practices, we have been blessed to watch our son heal from years of physical ailments and suffering.

Many conditions and diseases we face today can be diminished or eliminated by changing how we view healthcare and choose to take care of ourselves both physically and emotionally. Physically speaking, I have come to learn there are at least two very distinct and profoundly different schools of thought on healthcare. I have tried one way, modern medicine, for ten years. It was not working for my son. I decided to take a few steps to see where the second school of thought, holistic health, would take him.

I do have to say the holistic or more natural approach to medicine and prevention has been far more successful for my son than the typical or more common approach to treating disease. I will also say that five years ago I had absolutely no idea what the natural or holistic approach to medicine or disease was or how it could possibly help my son. I was beginning this dramatic change not knowing where to look or turn for assistance and guidance. I have been pleasantly surprised by the endless array of holistic therapies, practitioners, modalities, and resources that exist out there for all of us. These resources are in all of our communities and right at our fingertips. We just have to learn how to access them.

Frankie lived the first ten years of his life in and out of the pediatrician and specialist's office while being treated mainly for allergy and asthma symptoms. He was prescribed approximately 125 separate doses of inhalers, steroids, medications, and antibiotics over those same years to treat his symptoms. As we later came to understand, Frankie's yeast overgrowth (Candida) and the disruption of his normal body flora was due to years of continued antibiotics, inhalers, oral steroids, poor diet, and an overworked immune system. He lived for more than ten years with a body that was fighting hard to stay healthy. His symptoms were a continuous and outward sign that his body was not in proper balance. Candida, a poor diet, and exposure to too many man-made chemicals in food and the environment all preyed on his young body. Disease and illness found a comfortable home in which it wreaked havoc and chaos for years. His symptoms mimicked those of asthma and he was receiving medical treatment in a manner that did not serve him. I was trying to help him the only way I knew how - the medical, antibiotic, and medication way.

I helplessly watched this beautiful child become progressively more ill with not only an increase in symptoms, but with an increase in severity and duration of symptoms as well. I silently and ignorantly complied with his doctors until finally, with strong conviction and angered motivation, I said, "enough is enough." I finally took control of his health care in March of 2009. I helped him make some drastic changes to what he was putting into his body. In the five years since I began educating myself on nutrition, the digestive system, antibiotic overload, healthy eating, and the dangers of our nation's current food supply, he has come off all asthma and allergy medications. He has also been to the pediatrician only twice for sick visits and both visits were back in 2010. He has not been back to the pediatrician in over four years because of allergy or asthmatic symptom(s). The diagnosis of asthma has also been removed from his permanent record by his new pediatrician after a specified time period of no sicknesses. He is no longer dependent on antibiotics, medications, steroids, inhalers, nebulizer machines, and a team of specialists to treat his long list of daily symptoms. He is now a healthy active sixteen year old boy!

Through research, perseverance, and an open mind I have come to understand and accept some very important concepts and ideas that have changed our lives hopefully forever and already for the better.

1. Antibiotics: The overuse of antibiotics is hurting our children (and us for that matter) more than we are talking about or fully understand. You don't hear much about this extremely important topic in "mainstream America" and I have to wonder why.

Do you know what happens to our bodies, specifically our digestive systems, when we take an antibiotic? The digestive system plays such a vital role in all aspects of our overall health. I knew very little about how it worked and ways I could improve or enhance its functioning. Maintaining good digestive health is one of the key elements to a healthy body. I did not have a concrete, working knowledge of what was happening to my children every time they were given an antibiotic to treat an illness or symptom. I did not understand how dynamic the entire human body is and how given the right nutritional and emotional support, it can heal itself. Antibiotics are sometimes recommended and needed to help with a medical condition, illness, or disease. However, I am talking about the prescribing of medicine and antibiotics that came to be routine for my son. I am also referring to the overprescribing of medications and antibiotics for all children at a time in their life when their bodies are growing and developing.

One potential side effect from the use of inhalers and steroids individuals use in the treatment of asthma or other medical conditions is a condition called Candida. Candida is an unwelcome yeast overgrowth that begins in the digestive system. If left untreated, Candida has the potential to spread symptoms to other parts of the body and can cause hundreds of acute and chronic symptoms in a "healthy" person. It has the potential to fester, stealth-like in the body. It also has the potential to cause a whole host of physical and emotional symptoms that are often times misdiagnosed by the medical community. These symptoms will inevitably get worse if left untreated. This was also the case for my son.

The undiagnosed chronic yeast infection that is more and more common in our children today is silently and painfully hurting them. The antibiotics we are so willingly administering to our children at the first sign of a symptom or sickness is upsetting the normal flora in their bodies. Normal flora refers to the digestive environment in a person's body. Both Candida and the disruption of the normal bacteria in Frankie's digestive tract were silently and painfully causing damage for years. For as much as he had to endure physically through the years, he is fortunate. Most people go their entire lives not knowing that Candida and an unhealthy digestive system are causing or contributing to illness, disease, general ill-feelings, and emotional ups and downs.

2. Food Supply: I have come to understand that food—specifically the chemicals and toxins added to this food—that we are knowingly and unknowingly giving to our children are loaded with processed sugars, corn, gluten and soy derivatives, fatty oils, chemicals, growth hormones, antibiotic and pesticide residue, genetically engineered organisms, and is grown in soil containing hazardous fertilizers. Some of these same foods contain artificial flavors, colors, and preservatives. We are giving our children foods that are full of man-made or synthetic chemicals and toxins. Not only are we not providing the right foods for our children, but the ingredients used in the mass production of that very same food has the potential to worsen physical and behavioral symptoms in all of us. I know we all want to provide our children with healthy food choices. I think if we had a better understanding of exactly how the food industry has changed, especially with regard to the mass production of food, we would think twice about what we are actually serving our children at the kitchen table and in their lunch bag. Our children are exposed to chemicals everywhere. At some point these toxins will have a negative effect on their overall health. We live in a toxic world! We must gain an understanding of how to reduce our children's daily exposure to these harmful ingredients. You must become or continue to be an advocate on behalf of your children as you navigate your way through the barrage of marketing and advertising of food products by the gigantic companies who stand to profit financially from your family.

3. Health issues facing our children today: It seems perplexing to me that while some individuals would say we live in one of the most advanced medical, educational, and agricultural country in the world, we are experiencing a dramatic increase in the number of children being diagnosed with asthma, ADHD, skin conditions, environmental allergies, food allergies, ADD, obesity, gastrointestinal disorders, cancers, diabetes, autism, behavioral problems, mental health concerns, and the list goes on and on. The question I ask is why? Why are these disorders, diseases, and conditions increasing at such alarming rates?

This country has the best educated doctors anywhere in the world with a medical community that is innovative and scientifically superior. I firmly believe doctors make a conscious choice to want to help people get better. They have spent many years and sacrificed much to earn the title of M.D. However, something is fundamentally missing. I do not solely blame the doctors for what I think is missing in the parameters of healthcare today. I believe one of the missing pieces to the medical model today is the holistic approach of medical prevention rather than disease control. Disease management was not working for my son. I changed the premise of my thinking and decided to pursue ideas and treatment plans that included the *elimination* of his symptoms. Maintaining or controlling his daily symptoms through medications, antibiotics, nebulizer machines, and steroids was no longer a viable option for Frankie. The treatment plans laid out by the doctors through the years did not work to assist him in balancing the numerous symptoms and illnesses he faced on a daily basis. I was in search of something better. I was in search of a treatment plan that would bring him freedom and good physical health without daily medications.

4. Holistic Care: By deciding to change my thought process about illness, a whole new world has opened up to my family. The holistic approach to patient care incorporates the mental, emotional, physical, and spiritual health of an individual. Holistic health connects the mind, body, and spirit. It also includes a wide range of therapies and philosophies that focus on the prevention of illness. Holistic care is a lifestyle choice. A generic definition of the word "holistic" taken from the Merriam Webster dictionary is "relating to or concerned with wholes or with complete systems rather than the analysis of, treatment of, or dissection into parts". A holistic approach to health looks at the WHOLE person.

There was no roadmap that I was aware of for me as I began this newfound journey into the world of holistic care. I turned to holistic treatments as a last ditch effort to help my son. I had absolutely no idea what I was doing or if he would benefit from the changes I was about to implement in my home. I do know the gradual disappearance of his life-long symptoms and numerous diagnoses laid the foundation for my on-going journey into holistic health.

This new holistic world (preventative care) for my family consists of: understanding and implementing proper nutrition through foods, vitamins and supplements, use of homeopathic remedies, ridding or reducing our house of chemicals, and eliminating antibiotics and maintenance medications. We also now incorporate acupuncture, are learning about and maintaining better emotional support, identifying daily stressors and eliminating or better understanding those stressors, an introduction to meditation and yoga practices, and a desire to simplify my family's daily life. It is my belief that one cannot travel the path of life and truth if the body, mind, and spirit are not alive, awakened, and aware. Am I there yet? Without hesitation, the answer is a resounding no. I may never get there. Isn't it a pleasant thought though that good health, peace of mind, and a free spirit are ours for the taking if we so choose?

5. Education: If we can educate this generation of children on these specific and important topics, not only will their life expectancy increase, but their quality of life will increase as well. I am talking about a fundamental change in how we approach and educate our children about food, medications, disease, nutrition, the commercialism of society today, and the importance of healthy and simple living.

It is no longer enough to discuss and educate our children about the food pyramid or food plate. We must take it a step further and delve into some of these issues that will be explored in the coming pages with an open mind. The federal government and its regulatory agencies have decided it is their job to intervene into the protection and oversight of our food supply and medical care in order to protect us. However, corporations are poisoning our food supply with chemical after chemical and we are experiencing an increase in diseases at an exceptionally high rate. There is mounting research to suggest there is a direct correlation between the chemicals being added to our foods and our overall health. In the end, it is all of us who will suffer and pay the consequences. A systemic failure has occurred in this country. Yet, we have the power to change its course by directing our attention to several important and often overlooked topics. How can we inform people of the need for change? One person and one story at a time!

CHAPTER 2
Through the Years:
Frankie's Story

*"Out of suffering have emerged the strongest souls;
the most massive characters are seared with scars."*
-Kahlil Gibran

Years...It has been years of doctor visits, invasive and non-invasive medical testing, consultations, procedures, specialists, waiting rooms, thousands and thousands of dollars in medications and co-payments, doctor inadequacies, and of specialists not taking the time or having the knowledge to help my son. It has been years of allergy testing, nebulizer machines, inhalers, maintenance medications, rescue medications, oral steroids, blood tests, CT scans, chest X-rays, breathing tests, numerous diagnoses, antibiotics, and medications. It has been years of consoling and providing comfort to a child who has been repeatedly poked, prodded, scanned, and stuck.

Years...It has been years of pediatricians and specialists medically diagnosing my son with asthma (unspecified with exacerbation), exercise induced asthma, thrush, sleep development problems, gastroenteritis, strep throat, bronchitis, upper respiratory infections, croup, migraines, exercise induced headaches, reactive airway disease, rhino rhea, chronic sinus infections, allergies, non-allergic rhinitis, pneumonia, hay fever, laryngitis, ear infections, pharyngitis, chronic cough, cough-variant asthma, viruses, colds and flu's, psychological cough, psychological throat clearing, mucus problems, mild acid reflux, mild non-acidic reflux, laryngeal reflux, vocal cord damage, and allergic rhinitis. Some of these diagnoses were given to him over and over again through the years. He has also undergone surgery to have tubes placed in his ears and his adenoids have been removed as recommended by his doctor.

Years...It has been years of missed parties, missed family gatherings, missed sporting activities, missed school, missed or interrupted vacations, and missed opportunities that my family—my son specifically—will never be able to get back. It has been years of symptoms that have only gotten worse as he has grown. It has been years of a child not feeling well with no answers. This has always been the most challenging and heartbreaking part of this journey. I knew my child was sick. I observed his daily symptoms like no one else and often verbalized to his doctors where he was in what I called an "episode." Looking back on the situation, his young body was dictating the length and severity of an "episode" with complete disregard to the medical treatment he had received and to the nutritional diet I was or wasn't providing for him. These episodes usually started and ended with the same symptoms no matter what medicine or antibiotic the doctors gave him. Once the initial symptoms began to emerge, I would ready myself, him, the family, and the house. I would clean the house in an attempt to eliminate asthma triggers. I knew for the next few weeks he would be sick. My time was always focused on preventing an episode or helping him through an episode. I was failing miserably because seventy five percent of the time I was struggling to do both.

Years...It has been years of watching my child participate in sports struggling to keep up, to sick too fully participate, and overcome with sheer exhaustion at the end of the activity. I cannot count the number of times I sat on the sideline of a soccer game, ice hockey game, or track meet and watched my son struggle to run. Not because he was having an asthma attack and having difficulty breathing, but because he was congested, feverish, coughing, and sick. I could look at his sweet face and know he did not feel well. It always amazed me that he somehow was managing to stay active. I believe God knew exactly what He was doing when He gifted this child with a fierce competitive spirit. It is, without question, what carried him through this long, sometimes dark experience.

Because his body was weaker than the other boys he competed against, he would take much longer to recover physically. He suffered in silence. I truly did not know if the constant running and exercise was hurting him even further. (As I later learned, exercise for someone with Candida is especially important.) He was able to get through most days without anyone ever knowing how bad he really felt. He went to school unless he was at his worst. A few times the school had to call me to come pick him up because his coughing was disrupting the entire class. This was while he was on all of his asthma medications. His cough was the most visible outward physical symptom the world around him observed. However, there were so many more. It was like a prison for him and the rest of the family. Frankie seldom talked about how he felt physically. He just trudged on with his day doing the very best he could. It was his and our norm. It was all he knew and my heart broke for him.

Years...It has been years of frustration, worry, anger, patience and impatience, heartache, stress, sadness, and discontentment. That is how I felt. Now imagine how my son felt. His physical problems were exhausting. As a mother who was doing everything humanly possible to help her son, his symptoms left both of us physically and emotionally drained.

"Don't worry. He is not contagious. He has asthma." I must have said that exact phrase a thousand times in my lifetime to people who got a firsthand glimpse of Frankie's symptoms. I use to say it to friends, family, store clerks, teachers, strangers, and coaches. I would try to reassure them that these symptoms were just part of who he was and he couldn't get them sick. I felt helpless and scared for my son.

Years...It had been years of the same symptoms repeating themselves several times a year or never really going away at all. How must it feel to wake up each morning not knowing what the day will bring to a child who is constantly battling symptoms that no doctor or medication is able to help with? It was a feeling of complete helplessness and hopelessness. The symptoms we are talking about he has had for a lifetime. Too many years had passed with no improvement for my son. What would his future be if I could not help him get these symptoms under control? If I had decided to stay on the same medical path, I believe somewhere down the road he was going to be in trouble with his health. The quality of those years would have been the same as the past: antibiotics, medications, doctor visits, new diagnoses, and new illnesses. Missed parties, missed school, and interrupted vacations and family activities would have continued as well. His symptoms were getting worse and new symptoms and diagnoses were emerging as the years progressed. Besides the physical symptoms and ramifications of not feeling well, the emotional toll was increasing the older he became. There had to be a better system in place other than continuing to push medications that have done little to nothing to reduce the severity or duration of his lifelong symptoms.

Years... 2009 is the year I began to challenge the doctors, specialists, and medical community for an answer. This is the year I took a different path in regard to the medical treatment for my son. My defining moment came during one particular visit with his pediatrician at the beginning of 2009. This visit awoke the advocate inside of me. This moment was the absolute turning point for me as a mother in regard to my son's health. I remember feeling angry because I felt like his pediatrician was not hearing or listening to my concerns about his health. She told me that I was part of the problem with the healthcare crisis in this country. I was directly told I was part of the problem because I was having him undergo unnecessary tests and procedures that are expensive and a waste of everyone's time and energy (2009 is the first time I began looking for answers outside of what his pediatricians or asthma specialists were telling me to do). Frankie had followed all of the treatment plans given to us by his doctors through the years with a limited positive outcome. I was still searching for conventional medical options for Frankie, but was unknowingly beginning the journey into alternative medicine and healing. His pediatrician's treatment plan was to continue pushing asthma medications, antibiotics, and steroids.

It was not just this pediatrician, but the pediatricians before her and all the specialists that Frankie had seen in his short lifetime. It was a systemic failure on the part of the medical profession and a complete lack of understanding on my part.

Frankie began taking medications at the age of one month old. He continued taking antibiotics and medications until finally when Frankie was ten years old I said, "No more. Something is wrong and you do not have the answers. I will do everything in my power to find those answers."

Frankie's doctor compounded my angered motivation by saying to the both of us that Frankie was part of the problem as well. She continued by telling Frankie directly that "he is not sick. He is a healthy ten year old boy with asthma." I was disheartened by the manner in which his pediatrician spoke to him on what would be our last visit with her. I would describe her communication to us as arrogant and self-serving. She looked at my son and in a demeaning and authoritative voice told him "You are not dying, you do not have cancer, and you need to go outside while I talk with your mother." I don't know about you, but I could not have imagined that any pediatrician would look a ten year old child in the eyes, scold them, and tell them they do not have cancer when that is the farthest diagnosis from anyone's mind. For a few days after that Frankie would ask me if he was more ill than he thought or that I was telling him. How can a woman who dedicates her professional life to the health of young people treat a patient—a child—in such a negative way? Isn't it a doctor's fundamental philosophy to do no harm to a patient? I explained to her that I needed a doctor who would be my partner in trying to get Frankie healthy. The look on her face immediately told me we would never work together for the good of my son. I knew that Frankie would never again walk into her office. We were not partners, nor would we ever work together to assist Frankie in getting his "asthmatic" symptoms under control. She was the expert and I was "just" the parent. It appeared to me that she was just as frustrated as I was in that moment. She was trying to help him based on her knowledge of the human body and education.

There was never any clarity as to why she never looked for yeast infections that occur in children who use steroids and inhalers. There was no ongoing dialogue with his pediatrician about the underlying cause of his symptoms. I'm sorry, I take that back. She conveyed to me several times he had asthma. End of discussion! That answer was not good enough for me anymore given his bodily response to years of asthma medications. It took a long time for me to understand and accept that she was coming from a different point of view. This pediatrician was transferring her own world experience and education onto her patient, my son. In her decision to dismiss my concerns, she was unknowingly hurting him. It was time to find another pediatrician.

The more I thought about it and as I began my research for this book, I have come to understand that the medical community has not taken an in-depth look at the issue of Candida (chronic yeast infection) as a result of antibiotics or foods. It is my hope as more and more information, research, studies, and personal stories come out about this very important topic there will be a change in perspective on how doctors medically treat their patients. One of the changes that need to be implemented is to stop treating bodily illnesses or diseases separately and exclusively. Is it possible to look at the body as an entire entity with many moving parts? Medications certainly have their place in helping to cure physical illness and disease, but we are undereducated as to how powerful our bodies are in fighting disease, symptoms, and chronic and acute illnesses when given the right education and support.

In March of 2009 Frankie was diagnosed with Candida in the esophagus by the gastrointestinal doctor he was now seeing for his symptoms. Three months later he was diagnosed with Candida in the Larynx by the Mayo Clinic in Minnesota. It is evident to me over the years that the doctors completely overlooked, and now dismissed, a diagnosis of Candida and a significant imbalance of the normal flora in his digestive tract. I think it is interesting to note where Frankie struggled the most in terms of his symptoms is exactly where the yeast infections were medically confirmed. All of his doctors were downplaying the significance of Candida which had me extremely confused. I, on the other hand, was hopeful. I thought I might finally have the answer I have been searching for in regard to my son's health. Did I want him to have this diagnosis? Absolutely not, but it gave me hope that we were on the right track. I began to learn more about what Candida was but still needed to figure out how to rid his body of it for good. This is when I realized I was on this medical journey by myself. It was up to me to educate myself on asthma and its symptoms,

Candida and its symptoms, and anything else that was presented to us along the way. This was the year I would begin to free my son from illness and a dependency on doctors and medications. I was determined to find a way to uncage the beautiful qualities and traits that had been hidden or lying dormant beneath a haze of medications, antibiotics, and sickness.

Years...It has been almost five years since our family made the switch from conventional, modern medicine and a poor diet to a more holistic approach to life. The fog of sickness, continuous antibiotics, and maintenance medications has lifted. By changing Frankie's diet, ridding my house of as many chemicals as possible, and providing his body with the proper nutritional support through diet, vitamins, and other supplements, he is now a physically healthy child. There are no physical restrictions for him. I no longer need to cart a nebulizer machine with us on our travels in case he starts wheezing, Advil in case he gets a headache, or inhalers to prevent or treat an asthmatic attack. There are no more sick visits to the pediatrician or specialists. I do not have to spend my time removing allergy triggers from the house or preparing everyone else for an "episode." He does not miss school, vacations, special events, sporting activities, or just hanging out with his friends because he is sick. The worry, frustration, anger, and hopelessness concerning my son's physical discomfort have diminished. Frankie serves as a role model for understanding and accepting that change is possible no matter what age you are in life.

One of the lessons I have come to understand is that your relationship with your pediatrician is of vital importance. You are an equal partner in the medical treatment of your child! If you are not a partner, it is time to find another doctor! I cannot be clearer about this issue. If your questions and concerns regarding the health of your child are not being heard and considered, it is time to find a doctor that makes you a partner in the health of your child. Do not get me wrong, the doctor is the medical expert. However, you are the expert in regard to your child. Your questions, concerns, and input are a vital component of any and all non-emergency treatment plans for your child.

I believe in my heart there are wonderful pediatricians all over this country. You have to do some research and find the one that meets your family's needs. No one is going to take better care of your family than you. Find a pediatrician who takes the time to answer your questions and who you believe has the right educational background to best treat your child. There are several factors to consider when choosing a pediatrician. Some of those factors have been outlined below. Take the time to think about and research what you want in a pediatrician. It is important to consider who is managing your family's health.

PRACTICAL THINGS TO CONSIDER WHEN CHOOSING A PEDIATRICIAN OR PEDIATRIC GROUP:

- Verify insurance coverage.
- What is the distance of the office from your home?
- What are the office hours? Is the office open on the weekends?
- How would you rate the cleanliness of office?
- Is the pediatrician board certified? What other educational credential and training has he or she obtained?
- Do they have a specialty?
- How easy is it to make an appointment?
- What is the average wait time for appointments?
- How would you rate the friendliness of staff including receptionists and nurses?
- Obtain references from family and friends.
- Does the office call you back in a timely manner?
- What type of support staff is in the office and what are their credentials?
- What hospital(s) is the pediatrician affiliated with?

Other things that you should consider when selecting a pediatrician for your family:

COMMUNICATION:

- Will your pediatrician advise you of all the necessary information in regard to immunizations, developmental milestones, and the latest studies and concerns on a specific topic(s)? Instead of just being handed a fact sheet about a specific topic, I would look for someone who voices your concerns as a mother. For example, "I understand you have questions about the vaccine schedule. I did too when my children were young. This is the information that I found helpful, etc." If the pediatrician cannot take thirty seconds to validate your concerns or questions about your child, it should be an indicator or red flag for you.

FAITH:

- Are you given any special consideration in regard to your religious or spiritual beliefs as it relates to vaccines, circumcision, and breast feeding?

BEDSIDE MANNER:

- Pay special attention to the pediatrician's verbal and nonverbal mannerisms. Is he or she friendly? Do they remember your name without looking at the file? Does he or she engage the child in conversation depending on age? Does he or she make your child feel comfortable and ease their anxiety? Do they tell your child specifically what they are going to do during the exam? Does the pediatrician engage in conversation about your concerns? Do they seek input from you? Are you able to ask questions?

COMMITMENT:

- How long does the pediatrician spend with you and how informative is that time? Your time is just as valuable as any pediatrician's. You should not feel rushed. Your pediatrician should be committed to your child's overall health. Spending time with your child shows a sense of commitment.

NUTRITION:

- How does your pediatrician feel about the use of supplements and vitamins (I am not just talking about a fruit flavored, once a day chewable vitamin)? Are there any holistic approaches to medicine that they utilize in the office? Does the pediatrician engage in or talk about your child's diet and what you can do to help boost their immune systems naturally? Do they talk about chemicals and how to reduce them?

ANTIBIOTICS:

- What is the general guideline your pediatrician uses when dispensing medications or antibiotics? If you do not want your children to be given antibiotics for every illness, will your pediatrician provide alternative recommendations or suggestions? Do they suggest taking prebiotics and probiotics after antibiotics to promote good bacterial growth? Ask about how the digestive system is disrupted when an antibiotic is administered. What kind of answer do you get?

KNOWLEDGE:

- Does your pediatrician have a working knowledge that includes not only a medical background, but one of common sense, courtesy, respect, and ideas on different ways to treat illness? Do they offer alternative approaches to the health of your child?

I will also suggest to you that while it is extremely important to find a pediatrician that you feel meets your family's needs, it is equally important to consider other preventative healthcare measures to ensure your family's health. If you are interested, a good starting point would be to find and talk with a homeopathic practitioner in your immediate area. They are an excellent resource and can provide you with much information. If you are interested these resources can be found on page 258-259.

CHAPTER 3
The Journey:
Symptoms and Medications

"The superior doctor prevents sickness; the mediocre doctor attends to impending sickness; the inferior doctor treats actual sickness."

—CHINESE PROVERB

This chapter focuses on Frankie's medical journey from a typical medical approach and from the beginnings of a holistic approach toward taking care of his body. It is my hope this will assist you in better understanding his medical path to date and that it will help lay the foundation for a change in your child's or your own medical treatment plan. I have pieced his timeline together through medical records and his prescription history. I have missed a few things along the way. However, it is my absolute best calculation based on all of the medical records that I have been able to obtain to date.

FRANKIE'S PHYSICAL SYMPTOMS:

- Throat cough
- Increase in mucus in back of throat
- Begins snorting, clearing throat increases, and congestion begins in throat and nose
- Mild hoarseness when speaking
- Usually will not be able to produce mucus by blowing nose
- Begins to not feel well
- Signs of lethargy
- Hoarseness of voice becomes moderate to severe
- Cough moves from throat to chest
- Fatigue and exhaustion
- Irritability, moodiness, and emotional ups and downs
- Interrupted sleep patterns due to cough and kicking of legs
- Night-time coughing
- Fevers
- Wheezing
- Cough turns into a dry, hacking, and non-stop cough that could last weeks
- Dark circles under eyes
- Lack of appetite (picky eater who loves sugar, carbohydrates, and processed foods)
- Debilitating headaches (usually during or after sports)
- Mental fogginess, lack of concentration, forgetfulness, and inattention
- Postnasal drip
- Molluscums (viral type wart)
- Gas, diarrhea, and constipation

I encourage you, if you are concerned about your child's health, to begin a daily journal documenting symptoms, diagnosis, and treatment plans. You can also include foods eaten, drinks consumed, weather, and behavior. You may be able to detect a pattern that has otherwise gone unnoticed. I compiled two notebooks that chronicled an entire year of his daily life and symptoms.

Here is an excerpt from a journal I used to write down Frankie's daily habits. This is also around the time I began to search for clarity and a better understanding regarding his health.

Example: Friday, March 6, 2009

Peak flow meter readings (asthma tool) are 260 and 300. (These readings are relatively normal and depend on which reference you are using as a guide).
Medications include: Pulmicort (twice daily), Astelin (twice daily), and Prilosec.

Foods include: bacon, waffles with syrup, peanut butter sandwich, pretzels, apple, fruit snack, organic licorice stick, combos, fried shrimp, strawberries, and bread.

Frankie complained of headache and not feeling well after his soccer game. He has lots of throat clearing. He was unable to fully participate in soccer game.

Frankie's Medical Timeline

Year	Number of Sick Visits	Medical Diagnosis	Medications
1999	9	7	6
2000	12	13	10
2001	10	12	16
2002	9	8	20
2003	10	11	13
2004	1	limited documentation	6
2005	limited documentation	limited documentation	2
2006	4	7	10
2007	9	7	15
2008	7	5	8
	71	70	106

Not included in the above doctor prescribed medication list are the over the counter medications and "other" things I have done over the years to help minimize Frankie's "asthmatic" symptoms at home. These measures were done continuously and multiple times.

OVER THE COUNTER MEDICATIONS & PREVENTATIVE MEASURES DONE AT HOME TO ALLEVIATE SYMPTOMS

- Mucinex
- Vicks Vapor Rub
- Daily children's chewable vitamin
- Advil and Motrin (many bottles)
- Nasal saline rinses (These were used hundreds of times during a course of approximately two years)
- Humidifier/vaporizer
- HEPA air cleaners in most rooms of the house
- Allergy-free bedding
- Air quality evaluations for home
- Yearly air duct cleanings
- Expensive air and heating filters
- Benadryl
- Triaminic Cough Syrup
- Delsym Cough Suppressant
- Robitussin- DM
- Daily food/weather logs
- Daily peak flow meter readings (asthma tool)
- Oscillococcinum (homeopathic remedy)
- Breathe Right Nasal Strips
- Samples of different medications and nasal sprays from doctor's offices

---

It is mindboggling to me as I began researching his medical abyss that not one doctor in ten years had an alarm bell go off in his or her head. WARNING! WARNING!

WARNING! What are we as medical professionals doing to positively enhance the health of this child? Why is it taking a mother to sound the alarm so to speak? I am done hitting the snooze button. I am not an expert, but I can tell you my son's medical abyss was not only disheartening, it was also completely unnecessary. How do I know my son's medical abyss was completely unnecessary? Toward the end of 2009 I changed my approach to disease, symptoms, and illnesses. With this change came a decrease and a progressive disappearance of disease, symptoms, and illnesses. They slowly went away!

Year	Number of Sick Visits	Medical Diagnosis	Medications
2009 (Jan.-July)	13	10	10

I separated 2009 from the rest of the above medical chart because it was toward the end of this year that my son began a more holistic approach to treating his symptoms. It was during the beginning of 2009 Frankie was feeling his worst. He was being seen by his pediatrician, an ENT, an asthma specialist, and now a gastrointestinal specialist. At my insistence and with the approval of one of his doctor's, Frankie came off his maintenance medications for asthma in March. We also spent three days at the Mayo Clinic in Minnesota to have a thorough evaluation of his symptoms. I felt like somebody was missing something in regard to my son's health. The visit to the Mayo Clinic still left me in search of answers for Frankie. I was disappointed with the outcome because in the end they diagnosed him with the same medical conditions as before. There was, however, another diagnosis of Candida that I discussed earlier. There is the Candida diagnosis again!

I made the decision for Frankie to begin seeing a homeopathic practitioner in August of 2009. I had very limited understanding about this type of approach to treating the human body. Would it work? Is this "junk" medicine? How does it work? What have I gotten my son into? Am I wasting my time and money on something I am not sure will help Frankie? What type of education or knowledge of the human body does this man have? Is he qualified? I was completely unsure of the right path for Frankie, but listened to my gut instinct which told me to go for it despite my hesitancy. Frankie had nothing to lose in regard to his health. It couldn't be any worse than what he had already experienced right? The homeopathic practitioner began by taking a full medical history. He slowly replaced medications and antibiotics with different vitamins, natural supplements, and homeopathic remedies based on Frankie's unique needs.

Year	Number of Sick Visits	Medical Diagnosis	Medications
2009 (Aug.-Dec.)	2	2	3

The above chart highlights the progression of change in Frankie's physical reaction to replacing antibiotics, medications, and an unhealthy diet with our growing and changing plan on treating the body from a holistic perspective.

I am glad I listened to my intuition or "gut" instinct. Over time his body began to improve! You can note the decrease of antibiotics and medications that were needed to help with his on-going symptoms. As the symptoms began to dissipate, so did the need for doctor appointments and medications. Frankie worked with this practitioner for approximately seven months. As the days, weeks, and months went by I could slowly see some positive changes physically and emotionally for him. However, he continued to have symptoms, just not as severe or debilitating. I knew from my research that a nutritionally rich diet would help enhance his body's ability to find its proper balance and optimal level of functioning. I wanted someone who would work with me from a nutritional point of view. I continued on with my quest and found a practitioner based in Florida who specializes in the treatment of Candida from a natural or holistic approach. We began working with him in June of 2010. Little did I know at the time, but without question, God had sent me an angel! My prayers for Frankie were being answered by a man that I had never met, nor have I met to this day.

At his request three different stool samples were sent to a lab for processing. All three results revealed that he had significant issues with Candida overgrowth (this was the third time in less than one year that Frankie was given this diagnosis). The results also showed he had a very high or toxic level of a normal kind of bacteria in the body called Klebsiella pneumoniae. Klebsiella pneumoniae is a type of bacteria that is usually found in the intestines or feces of humans and rarely causes a person to become sick. Just like the name sounds, it can cause pneumonia and affects the lungs. Hmmm. Could it be this bacteria, Klebsiella pneumoniae, that Frankie tested positive for at a very high or toxic level has been affecting his lungs for years? Frankie's test results also showed he did not have enough of certain good bacteria in his digestive system to fight the bad bacteria and chronic yeast infections. His immune system was working hard to fight off the fungus and bad bacteria in his body that it became over-whelmed and began to slowly break down creating more symptoms year after year. It was a vicious, vicious cycle. In the end, his digestive system was a cesspool of waste and toxins that were slowly being exported to the rest of his body. This was leaving behind a child who was chronically sick and emotionally drained.

The Candida specialist devised a treatment plan that eliminated dairy, corn, enriched white flours, wheat, and sugar from his diet altogether. There was an eight or nine month period where he did not eat or drastically reduced foods that contained any of these ingredients. We also began making the switch from conventional foods to organic foods. As we eliminated certain foods, he also began a daily regimen of vitamins and supplements (both liquid and pill form) that were based on the results of the stool sample testing and specific to him. His new doctor began a five phase treatment plan. This new treatment approach focused on digestive balancing. His doctor also began the slow process of educating me on the body, proper nutrition, and the importance of nutrition as it relates to health. This process continues to this very day!

Part of the treatment plan that was laid out for Frankie included:

Phase I (Alkalize Phase): Our blood becomes acidic over time as a result of antibiotics, environmental pollutants, and processed foods. This phase begins to alkalize the blood which brings it back to its natural and healthy state. It is important to understand that our body naturally has acidic fluids to help with the breakdown of food and the elimination of waste. We are not trying to alkalize the body, but rather to alkalize the blood which is the lifeline to the rest of the body and its systems.

Phase II (Replace Phase): This phase consists of the replacement of deficient nutrients such as vitamins, minerals, and fatty acids. This phase also includes the replacement of enzymes and other digestive factors that are lacking or limited in the gastrointestinal tract.

Phase III (Re-inoculate Phase): This phase reintroduces prebiotics, probiotics, and key bowel nutrients to assist in creating a healthy balance of desirable micro flora in the GI tract. Prebiotics create a healthy environment in which bacteria can grow. A probiotic is beneficial bacteria needed to aid in balancing digestive wellness.

Phase IV (Regenerate and Repair Phase): This phase provides support for the healing and growth of the lining of the intestinal tract.

Phase V (Remove Phase): The final phase eliminates harmful bacteria, viruses, fungi, and parasites from the GI tract.

This is a simplistic explanation to this five step process. I invite you to learn more about this program by going to www.nationalcandidacenter.com.

Over the next year a significant and remarkable change occurred in regard to Frankie's body and health. The decrease in antibiotics went from an average of eleven prescriptions per year for ten straight years to zero! In about one year he went from almost a prescription a month for his entire life to *zero!* His body, with the right vitamins, natural supplements, and a dramatic change in his nutritional intake, was healing itself. His symptoms continued to disappear and the haze of sickness continued to lift.

It was also at this time I began to realize his body was not only infected with yeast, but it also needed time to heal and detoxify from years of medications, antibiotics, steroids, and what I would now consider an unhealthy diet (a kid diet or the Standard American Diet). I was beginning the process of transitioning him from a SAD (Standard American Diet) to a GLAD (Green, Living, and Alkalizing/Abundant diet). It is important to understand your child's symptoms or lack of symptoms may be different or pose no health issues today. An unhealthy digestive system has the potential to contribute too many of the conditions we see today in our youth and in adults as well.

What is homeopathic medicine?

Homeopathic medicine is a medical philosophy based on the idea that the body has the ability to heal itself. The focus of homeopathy is on stimulating the body's own natural healing properties. It is stated Homeopathy began around 1796 by a man named Samuel Hahnemann. Homeopathy uses small or diluted remedies to relieve symptoms. Homeopathic practitioners decide what remedies to use based on a specific rule of nature called the Law of Similars. This law states: "like cures like," or that a medicine can cure a sick person if it can cause similar sickness in a healthy person. Remedies are made from the elements found in nature including minerals and plant extracts. The basis of these natural remedies is diluted through altering the degree of its concentration to avoid creating side effects that can be disagreeable. The more a homeopathic remedy is diluted, the stronger the remedy.

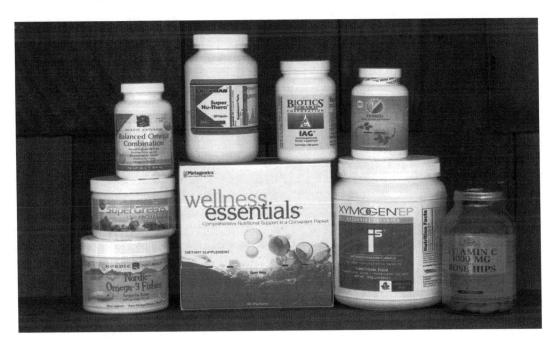

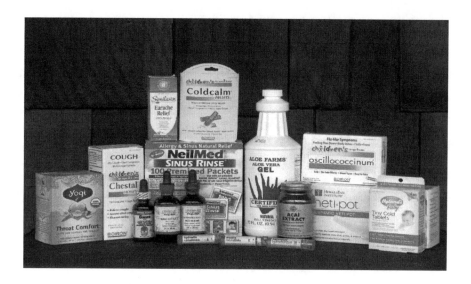

The years 2010, 2011, 2012, 2013, and 2014 prove to me yet again that taking care of your body naturally works. Frankie has succeeded in eliminating the number of doctor visits per year to one, his yearly exam. I could not be more proud of and happy for my son. He had the stamina, courage, strength, and fortitude to persevere in the face of radical change.

Year	Number of Sick Visits	Medical Diagnosis	Medications
2010	0	0	0
2011	0	0	2
2012	0	0	0
2013	0	0	0
2014	0	0	0

Somewhere toward what I thought was the end of this physical journey for Frankie, I began to discover and accept other holistic ideas and treatments for my entire family. As I reflect on his medical journey to date, it strikes me how simplistic in nature all of this is for us. By reducing chemicals, providing his body with the proper nutritional support, and allowing time for his body to heal, he overcame all of the physical limitations that have been with him since birth. WOW!

What I have come to better understand is that what our children are putting into their bodies is directly reflective of their overall health. We have to come to terms with the understanding and knowledge that our children live in a world full of chemicals and toxins. These chemicals and toxins are having negative, life changing effects on their overall physical, behavioral, and emotional health. Developing the knowledge and learning about the different ways children are exposed to chemicals on an everyday basis has given me the power to make the necessary changes to eliminate chemicals from my family's daily environment.

I now know what Frankie needs to do to maintain positive, physical health. The question is: Does Frankie want to continue with this lifestyle change? He is a teenager who wants to eat what everyone else is eating. He wants to be a "normal" child as defined by society today. His health has improved and is now in better balance. He is physically active, has more stamina, and can fully participate in school, sports, and life. His body has healed and it will be up to him to keep it that way. He has entered his teen years and has started high school. He will have to make choices independent of me that will affect his health and overall well-being. I will continue to support Frankie always, but I also know the time has come for me to give him wings to fly. I know he has the information, tools, and support to help him make good decisions now and in the future (Frankie's health continues to be maintained with limited outward physical symptoms. However, he continues to have significant digestive issues that require a focus on his diet and what he is choosing to eat. He is once again focusing on eating healthy for him. He is using vitamins, food, and other supplements to repair some of the damage that has been caused by returning to the typical American way of eating. Some of his physical symptoms have returned. He has become allergic to certain foods and will need to continue to monitor his consumption of these foods. In other words, his body cannot tolerate the Standard American Diet (SAD). His body cannot tolerate these foods on a consistent and ongoing basis. How he chooses to take care of himself will be something he has to decide for himself.).

John Ruskin once said, "We are not sent into this world to do anything into which we cannot put our heart." I put my heart and soul into helping Frankie overcome his physical limitations. By sharing part of our story, I hope I have inspired you about the possibility that change can happen and it can happen for you or your child if you so desire it. It is hard work and will require your commitment, determination, and positive attitude.

The remaining part of this book focuses on helping you understand what I had to learn the hard way regarding the unhealthy environment our children are living in today. It also explores some of the consequences this toxicity has on our overall health. How can our story help create a more safe, less toxic environment for your family? There are hundreds of ways to reduce the chemical and toxic overload our children are exposed to on any given day. I feel passionate about sharing the tips and information I have learned through research, books, holistic practitioners, articles, movies, and websites. I have also received valuable information from other people's personal experiences, stories, knowledge, and suggestions that have been passed on to me.

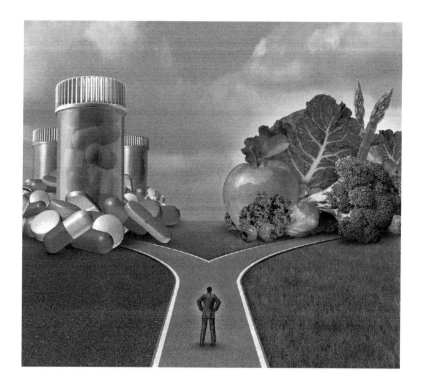

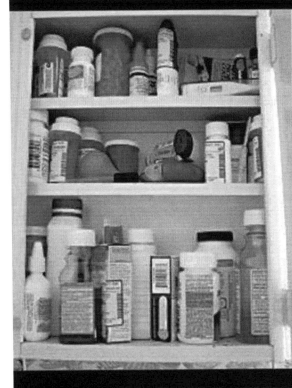
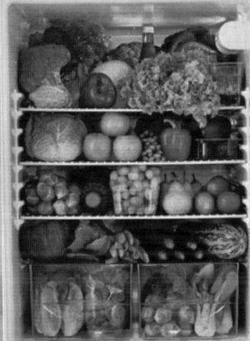
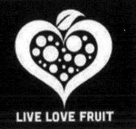

References

1. "Klebsiella pneumonia in Healthcare Settings", Accessed April 29, 2012, http://www.cdc.gov/HAI/organisms/klebsiella/klebsiella.html

2. The National Candida Center Program, Accessed April 24, 2014, http://www.national-candidacenter.com/candida-programs/

3. "What is Homeopathy", Accessed October 1, 2012, http://www.webmd.com/balance/guide/homeopathy-topic-overview

4. "Homeopathic Remedies: How are they Made"?, Accessed October 1, 2012, http://www.healthynewage.com/what-is-homeopathy.htm

5. "What is Homeopathy", Accessed October 1, 2012, http://nationalcenterforhomeopathy.org/content/learn-about-homeopathy

CHAPTER 4
The Body

"From the bitterness of disease man learns the sweetness of health."

-CATALAN PROVERB

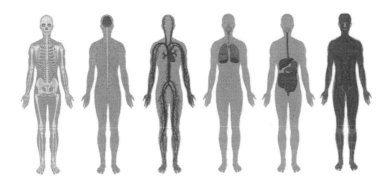

The average life expectancy of a particular group of people averages the number of years to be lived by a group of people born in the same year. The average life expectancy of an individual or group is affected by geographical location, age, sex, hereditary factors, race, occupation, and other factors. The average overall life expectancy in this country back in 1900 was 49.2 years and in 1950 it was 68.2 years. The life expectancy in 2011 was 78.5 years and in 2021 the average life expectancy will increase to 79.9 years. The average person born in the United States in six years will live to be almost eighty years old. My first thought is we must be doing something right. According to the Central Intelligence Agency (CIA), the United States of America ranks fiftieth in average life expectancy among 221 countries around the world. My second thought is this country, with all its advancement in technology and medicine, would be higher on this list. My concern is not merely the length of a person's life, but the *quality* of that life.

We now have the capabilities to extend life far beyond that which could have been imagined a generation ago (I am the recipient of these amazing capabilities and scientific advancements). We have gained powerful knowledge and a vast scope of treatment options to help us once we become sick. Medical and scientific innovations help to keep us alive for years or even decades. But, what is the quality of those remaining years? Modern medicine and scientific breakthroughs have paved the way for all future generations to live longer and longer. The more important information is that the quality of those years is being depleted and diminished. If we are going to live to be eighty years old, it is my hope those years be abundantly full of good health. Physically speaking, we need to begin extending the focus of modern medicine to include education, implementation, and direction on how to prevent disease rather than just trying to control it. I am referring to a more holistic treatment plan or modality for disease prevention and treatment. This concept is the most fundamental difference between the modalities of modern medicine and holistic health care.

The mind, body, and spirit are and will always be interconnected. Therefore, you cannot treat the body without understanding, learning about, and being aware of your mind and spirit. Healing (physical, emotional, or spiritual) is a result of understanding who you are on a profoundly deep and honest level. When you find the light within your soul, your truth can no longer hide. Finding your truth will enlighten your soul and bring about your freedom. Knowing who you are will increase the capacity to heal yourself, whatever the diagnosis. It is also worth mentioning that healing and curing is not the same thing. For example, a man may die of cancer because he could not be physically cured, but he may have healed the emotional or spiritual issues that have weighed him down for a lifetime. He is leaving this world in peace and WHOLE.

AS IT STANDS NOW IN THE UNITED STATES OF AMERICA:

- 1 out of every 15 people and 1 out of every 20 children are currently diagnosed with asthma. This is a 300 percent increase in the last twenty years.
- The rise in asthma was 42 percent in the United States from 1982–1992. The death rate rose 40 percent from 1982–1991.
- 10 percent of all children (5.5 million) in the United States are diagnosed with ADHD. This is an increase of almost 25 percent in four years.
- 1 out of every 400 to 600 children are diagnosed with type I diabetes. Diabetes affects 25.8 million people of all ages which is equal to 8.3 percent of the U.S. population.
- 1 out of 2 children will develop diabetes and 1 out of 3 adults will develop Type II diabetes.
- The rate of children diagnosed as obese has tripled in the last thirty years.
- 1 out of every 8 women will be diagnosed with an invasive form of breast cancer.
- 1 out of every 110 children and 1 out of every 70 boys will be diagnosed with an Autism Spectrum Disorder.
- Stroke affects more than 700,000 individuals annually in the United States (approximately one person every forty-five seconds). Someone in the United States dies every 3.3 minutes from a stroke.
- In the last twenty years there has been a 400 percent increase in food allergies. Approximately 3 million children in the United States have food allergies. Peanut allergies have doubled in children between1997-2002.
- Every year about 785,000 Americans will have their first heart attack. In 2006, heart disease caused 26 percent of all deaths and it is the leading cause of death for both men and women.

- 1 out of every 300 boys and 1 out of every 333 girls will develop cancer before their 20th birthday. Cancer is the number one cause of disease related death for children. In 2010, approximately 10,400 new cases of pediatric cancer were expected to be diagnosed. It should also be noted that while the incidence of invasive cancer in children has increased, the mortality rate has declined by as much as 50 percent.
- 1 out of every 3 people in this country will develop cancer in their lifetime.
- 1 out of every 5 people in this country will develop an autoimmune system disease.
- Recent findings estimate about 2 million people in the United States have celiac disease or about 1 in 133 people.

I believe one of the answers to the increase in diseases and conditions we are experiencing today is a direct result of, or made worse by, the environment in which we now live and that we have passed on to our children. We have become dependent on the medical and pharmaceutical industries. We have collectively and unconditionally accepted a flawed system of medical treatment for non-life threatening illnesses that leave us dependent on doctors and medications to sustain our lives. What would it take to become less dependent on doctors, pharmaceutical companies, and our own government? The answer is as simple as *Education* and *Personal Empowerment*!

I also believe parents might take the opportunity to consider making changes to their child's daily environment if they had the facts about antibiotic overload, toxins, chemicals in food, and the overload of other man-made or synthetic chemicals that are inundating our children's bodies on a daily basis and contributing to or causing disease and behavioral maladies.

Another separate and specific cause for concern for our children is the low-levels of radiation and electromagnetic energy being emitted from the electronic and wireless devices that are used on a daily and constant basis. This issue is a little off topic and is extremely important.

As our children enter the age of technology, we can now include the use of cell phones, computers, and "dirty electricity" as major potential health risks due to the low levels of radiation and electromagnetic energy being emitted from these devices.

Electromagnetic fields (EMF's) are a type of low-level frequency that is emitted from anything that is electronic and electrical in our culture today. The three different kinds of EMF's we need to be aware of are magnetic, electric, and radio frequency. More and more studies and research on these potential dangers are compelling parents to create safe boundaries for their children. The scientific evidence is growing and is a cause for concern and a watchful eye. If you want to learn more about EMF dangers, I suggest using Google to start your search.

Scientific studies are making the connection between tumors of all kind, an increase of brain tumors, headaches, cell and DNA damage, sleep disorders, and increased cancer risk as potential consequences to our overall health as a result of our daily exposure to radiation and electromagnetic energy sources. Other studies are looking at electromagnetic radiation and energy as aggravating and contributing factors to Parkinson's and Alzheimer's disease, chronic fatigue, brain fog and forgetfulness, leukemia, stress, fibromyalgia, heart problems, birth defects, and tinnitus to name a few.

We live in an age of technology. There is no way to avoid these devices. However, there are things you can do to lower your exposure to their negative effects. First, I would suggest you research this topic on your own. See what you find. I would also suggest not putting the phone to your ear, not using a Bluetooth ear piece (also emits radiation), and to limit putting phones in your pocket or carrying on you for extended periods of time. I ask you to consider powering down and turning off all electronics in your bedroom and your child's bedroom before going to sleep. Can you turn off or unplug most electronics in your house at the end of the day? If you use your cell phone as an alarm clock, can you put it in airplane mode or turn off the wireless connection? Can you power down the electronics you are not using during the day? How about putting your phone or wireless devices in airplane mode so they are not constantly searching for a wireless signal? Children have thinner skulls than adults which may make them more susceptible to the many and now better understood negative effects. Texting is a better option for all of us than constantly being on the phone. Use a corded phone where you can and purchase a headset that reduces radiation exposure. Can you be more mindful of your use of appliances and devices throughout the day?

There are meters that can be purchased or rented to test the EMF fields in your home. When looking to purchase an all-purpose meter, the TriField 100XE is the one I keep finding in my research as the best one due to its accuracy and cost ($120). If you have serious concerns that EMF's are causing health problems, contacting a professional trained in EMF reduction might prove helpful. Other devices that emit low levels of radiation or that have an electromagnetic fields of energy include: microwaves, alarm clocks, x-ray scanners, power lines, cordless phones, transformers, smart meters, electrical panels, household appliances, wireless routers; doorbells; and intercoms, cordless baby monitors, wireless internet connections, and wireless gaming systems.

This is an invisible problem that has the potential to create significant health consequences for all of us. It is another way that our bodies are being inundated with daily things that do not promote health and vitality. These devices help to break our body down over time and possibly contribute to a host of health issues. To learn more about cell phone danger, please go to http://products.mercola.com/blue-tube-headset/. Countries around the world are establishing guidelines and safer recommendations for cell phone use. They would not being doing this if there was not a cause for concern! For some reason our government, cell phone companies, and the telecom industry at large do not feel this issue is important enough to educate consumers. If these devices are on or near our bodies 24/7 and emit low levels of radiation and EMF's, how can we not begin to make some small connection to the health issues we are all facing today?

The power of your health and your child's health has to be in your hands. The federal government should not have the power or authority to mandate or dictate what you eat or what options are available to you medically. Our society and corporations are dictating what we eat, how much we eat, where we eat, and they are doing it with chemically produced, harmful foods. This generation's children are losing their childhoods and individual power to mass marketing and advertising, corporate greed, governmental inadequacies, societal overabundance, and a loss of personal freedom that is unparalleled at any other time in our country's history.

Until individuals and doctors start looking at disease prevention from a holistic perspective, we will continue to spend trillions of dollars a year to fight diseases instead of preventing them. In 2001, Americans spent $1.42 trillion dollars on health care. Thirteen years later, I would venture to guess that number has only increased. We will also continue to see a rise in the number of people using prescriptions drugs to maintain their health. We will not be in control of our health becoming more and more dependent on doctors, insurance companies, pharmaceutical companies, and sometimes our own government to provide the necessary treatments and medications to sustain our lives. We will live to be eighty years old, but what will the quality of those years be for us or our children?

The only conclusion I can come to is that we are missing a more natural and holistic approach to treating the human body. There has to be a better balance between health, prevention, and disease control. Please do not misunderstand what I am trying to say here. Medications and antibiotics have their place and have saved lives. Their advancement in the last fifty years has been incredible and life-saving. Our doctors and hospitals have the cutting edge technology to save a life that otherwise would not be saved. But, as a society we have become dependent on medicines and antibiotics for every day, non-life threatening ailments. We have lost sight of the importance of how dynamic our own bodies are in fending off disease and illnesses. We have to become the expert on our own health instead of the government, doctors, and pharmaceutical companies.

Through the power of education, we have the ability to redefine how we use the healthcare system in this country. It is also up to us to make a conscious decision to eliminate the toxins from our family's daily diet and environment. That is the good news! You can change your child's health for the better, create a less toxic environment for your family, and educate yourself on holistic principles if you so choose.

As I began this new holistic approach to eating and living, I also began the process of reeducating myself on the human body. Let's take a basic look at the major systems of the human body. These ten major systems make up the structural framework of each and every one of us. Each system has specific and important functions. It is important to remember that all the systems that make up the human body are interconnected. These systems rely on each other to perform their jobs and to function at their highest level. When there is a disruption in one system, it can lead to a disruption in another. In today's medical community we have specialists who are educated and concerned about one specific area of the body. These specialists treat one part of the body as a separate entity. If you look at the human body from a holistic perspective, all body systems are connected and function at their optimal or highest level when treated as a whole. Holistic health treats the body, not just the symptom.

The Major Systems of the Human Body:

1. Skeletal System: The main role of the skeletal system is to provide support and protection for the body. The skeletal system includes: bones, cartilage, tendons, and ligaments.

2. Muscular System: The main role of the muscular system is to provide movement. Muscles work in pairs to move limbs and provide the body with mobility.

3. Circulatory System: The main role of the circulatory system is to transport nutrients, gases, hormones, and wastes through the body. This system includes: the heart, blood vessels, and blood.

4. Nervous System: The main role of the nervous system is to relay electrical signals through the body. This system includes: the brain, spinal cord, and peripheral nerves.

5. Respiratory System: The main role of the respiratory system is to provide gas exchange between the blood and the environment. Oxygen is absorbed from the atmosphere into the body and carbon dioxide is expelled from the body. This system includes: the nose, trachea, and lungs.

6. Digestive System: The main role of the digestive system is to break down and absorb nutrients that are necessary for growth and maintenance. This system includes: the mouth, the esophagus, stomach, and the small and large intestines.

7. Excretory System: The main role of the excretory system is to filter out cellular waste, toxins, and excess water or nutrients from the circulatory system. This system includes: the bladder, urethra, and kidneys.

8. Endocrine System: The main role of the endocrine system is to relay chemical messages through the body. Many glands in the body secrete endocrine hormones. These glands include: the hypothalamus, pituitary, thyroid, pancreas, and adrenal.

9. Reproductive System: The main role of the reproductive system is to manufacture cells that allow reproduction. The reproductive system for a female is made up of the vagina, uterus, cervix, fallopian tubes, and ovaries. The reproductive system for a male is made up of the penis, testes, and seminal vesicles.

10. Immune System: The main role of the immune system is to destroy and remove invading microbes and viruses from the body. This system includes: the lymph nodes, vessels, and blood cells.

The next chapter in this book will focus on the one major body system that is often overlooked or downplayed as it relates to the overall health of an individual. While all systems are important individually and as a collective unit, the digestive system plays a vital role in our overall health.

References

1. Life Expectancy, Accessed May 23, 2011, http://www.data360.org/dsg. aspx?Data_Set_Group_Id=195

2. The World Fact Book, Accessed September 12, 2012, http://www.cia.gov/library/publications.the-world-factbook/rankorder/2012rank.html

3. The Allergy and Asthma Foundation of America. Asthma Overview, Accessed November 15, 2010, http://aafa.org/display.cfm?id=8&cont=5

4. Disease States Affected by MSG, Accessed April 25, 2014, http://www.msgtruth.org /disease.htm

5. "ADHD Is on the Rise: How to Use Nutrition to Treat Attention Deficit", Accessed November 16, 2010, http://www.huffington post.com/leo-galland-md/adhd-is-on-the-rise-_b_783381.html

6. American Diabetes Association. Diabetes Statistics, Accessed April 29, 2012, http://www.diabetes.org/diabetes-basics/statistics/

7. National Diabetes Information Clearinghouse. National Diabetes Statistics, 2011, Accessed April 29, 2012, http://www.diabetes.niddk.nih.gov/dm/pubs/statistics/dm_statistics.pdf

8. April 2010 Newsletter Top Preventative Measures For Quality Aging, Ann Boroch, Accessed April 25, 2014, http://www.annboroch.com/category/exercise-fitness/

9. Center for Disease Control. Childhood Obesity, Accessed November 17, 2010, http://www.cdc.gov/healthyyouth/obesity/

10. Breast Cancer.Org. Breast Cancer Statistics, Accessed December 3, 2010, http://www.breastcancer.org/symptoms/understand_bc/statistics.jsp

11. Autism Speaks. Accessed October 20, 2010, http://www.autismspeaks.org/

12. The University Hospital. Stroke Statistics, Accessed April 29, 2012, http//www.theuniversityhospital.com/stroke/stats.htm

13. Allergy Kids Foundation. "Defining Food Allergies", Accessed May 27, 2011, http://www.allergykids.com/denfining-food-allergies/defining-food-allergies/

14. CandleLighters.org. "Childhood Cancer Statistics", Accessed May 27, 2011, http://www.candle.org/who-we-are/childhood-cancer-facts

15. Inner Body. Select a Human Anatomy System Below to Begin:, Accessed April 25, 2014, http://www.innerbody.com/

16. Aron Bruhn, "Inside Human Body", New York: Sterling Publishing Company Inc., 2010.

17. Basic Anatomy – Organs and Organ Systems, "Basic Anatomy – Tissues and Organs", Accessed April 17, 2012, http://web.jjay.cuny.edu/~acapri/NSC/14-anatomy.htm

CHAPTER 5
pH Balance and
the Digestive System

"Digestion, of all the bodily functions, is the one which exercises the greatest influence on the mental state of an individual."

JEAN ANTHELME BRILLAT-SAVARIN (1755-1826)

I believe it is fair to say this country is facing an epidemic of digestive illnesses directly related to the foods we eat and the way we live. While it is believed that the majority of your immune system is located in or around the digestive system, it is the digestive system that is one of the most overlooked systems in the human body. An imbalance in this system is responsible for the onset of the majority of health conditions plaguing Americans today.

The main idea or theme to keep with you as you navigate your way through this part of the book is that the digestive system plays a pivotal and defining role in every aspect of our overall health. When there is an unbalance in this system, the process of disease, inflammation, and illness begins. A disruption in this system can also adversely affect all the other systems of the human body. It is within this system that most disease begins for all of us. In order to understand why this is the case, it is important to have a general idea of how our digestive system works. The digestive system's main jobs are to take the foods we consume and convert them into the necessary nutrients we need to fuel our bodies. It is also responsible for the proper elimination of bodily waste. It is made up of the mouth (teeth, tongue, and glands), pharynx, esophagus, stomach, appendix, liver, gall bladder, pancreas, small intestine, large intestine, rectum, and anus. They all work together to breakdown, process, and eliminate the food we consume on a day to day basis. The Kidneys are also vital in helping to rid the body of toxins.

The digestive system is made up of acids (to break down the food), digestive hormones and enzymes, bacteria, and yeast. Ideally, the bacteria and yeast should work in harmony with one another, but this balance is often interrupted by antibiotics, processed foods, stress, chemicals and toxins, and lack of a nutrient rich diet. Due to the way most of us currently live our lives, the proper balance of bacteria and yeast in the digestive system erodes over time. This leaves the body in a state of acidity or toxicity.

Another very important concept to understand that connects the food we eat to our digestive system and overall health is the balance between alkaline and acid in our blood. This concept is referred to as the *pH balance*. The pH scale measures the acidity or alkalinity of a solution. pH refers to potential hydrogen. Some people believe the acceptance and understanding of this concept will revolutionize the way we treat people with disease. I also believe if we have a general understanding of how this pH scale works in regard to the foods we eat and how our bodies function, we have the potential to prevent and reverse disease on a new level.

pH Balance

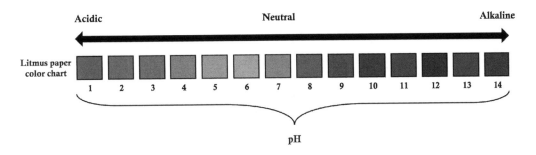

The pH scale is a numerical scale that ranges from 0–14. This scale is used to measure the acidity or alkalinity of a solution or substance. Basically, a neutral or 'basic" alkaline state is found in the middle of this scale. To the left are foods that are increasing in acidity and to the right are foods that are increasing in alkalinity. The easiest way to understand this scale and how it affects your body is to recognize that it is referring to an overabundance of acid as "bad" and a balanced or neutral alkaline state as "good." You can think of it as a teeter totter. You do not want this scale to tip too far one way or the other. For optimal health, we should seek the proper pH balance. Achieving the proper pH balance in your body is a delicate dance. This dance has the potential to physically change your life in a dramatic and positive way.

Your body's main goal to maximize health is to keep your pH level balanced. Balancing the pH level in your blood is your body's most important job and function throughout your lifetime. If your blood is acidic, your body will become deficient. You might experience: mental fogginess, headache, fatigue, skin conditions, PMS, allergies, irritability, digestive issues, sleep problems, colds and flu's, sinus problems, ear infections, muscle and joint pain, yeast infections, hypertension, bronchial ailments, and emotional disruptions such as anxiety, irritability, and depression. If acidity continues, you will not have enough oxygen available for your cells to stay healthy and to function normally. Fat cells are then formed to store the acidic waste. As a result, your body will possibly experience weight gain becoming a breeding ground for cancer cells, disease causing bacteria, fungus, viruses, and parasites.

The next step will be a development of plaque on your arteries causing, for example, inflammation or worse, heart disease. The last attempt by the body to restore the proper pH balance will be to take calcium from your bones. The progression of disease is clear. Different parts of your body require different pH levels. The pH level in your body can be measured in your blood, tissues, saliva, and urine. As a general rule, specific parts of your digestive system (example would be the stomach) will be a little bit more acidic than other parts of your body. The acid is required and is naturally produced to help in the process of elimination.

The best bodily indicator of how acidic (or unhealthy) our bodies are can be found in the blood. Just as our body temperature is maintained at 98.6 degrees Fahrenheit, our blood is ideally maintained at 7.365pH—very mildly "basic" or alkaline. Our blood only allows for a small shift in regard to the pH balance. The more acidic one's pH level in the blood, the more symptoms you have the potential to experience in the future. Over time, the acidity will lead to a fundamental breakdown in the body causing symptoms and disease to occur. Our bodies are working so hard to create a neutral or alkaline blood level that our tissues and organs are being deprived or depleted of vital nutrients. If the body is too acidic, it will automatically begin taking the nutrients from other areas such as your tissues, organs, and bones to compensate for this deficiency. The toxins are stored in the body and begin the process of decay and disease. As the acidity levels in the blood increase, the amount of necessary oxygen reaching the waiting cells is depleted and diminished. The cells in your body are struggling to survive and will begin to decay or die. The everyday maladies we don't think about as truly harmful to our overall physical well-being can take a further step toward the onset of diseases such as asthma, candida, high cholesterol, high blood pressure, type 2 diabetes, colitis, infertility, irritable bowel syndrome, cardiovascular diseases, multiple sclerosis, depression, Crohn's disease, insomnia, arthritis, poor memory, adrenal and thyroid problems, lupus, cancer, and so on.

WHAT IS CAUSING OUR BODIES TO BE MORE ACIDIC VS. ALKALINE?

- Unhealthy food choices including sugar, fast food, refined, packaged, and processed foods, unhealthy oils, contaminated meats, artificial flavorings and coloring, sweeteners, and preservatives.
- The overuse of antibiotics and medications.
- The lack of nutritional knowledge and understanding by parents and doctors.
- The onslaught of chemicals sprayed on fruits and vegetables including pesticides and chemical fertilizers. Genetically modified organism's (GMO's) is also a growing concern as it relates to the production and harvesting of the nation's fruit and vegetable supply. As new DNA is introduced during the process of genetic modification, the end result is that new proteins are added to the foods. Many individuals' immune systems cannot identify these new proteins and inflammation is created.
- Heavy metals found in vaccines, commercially farmed corn, water, and dental fillings.
- Unclean water sources
- Environmental toxins and pollution
- Lack of exercise and sleep
- Stress

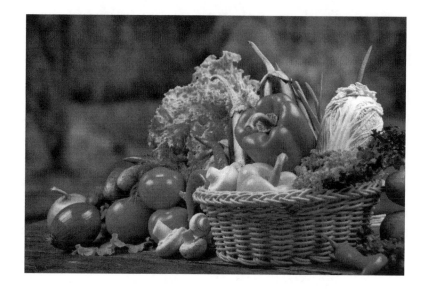

The Seven Most Alkalizing Foods

Kale

Cucumber

Broccoli

Spinach

Avocado

Celery

Bell Pepper/Pepper

The Top 10 Water-Rich Foods

Cucumber

Tomato

Carrots

Spinach

Broccoli

Watercress

Watermelon

Celery

Lettuce

Grapefruit

WHAT ARE SOME THINGS THAT I CAN DO TO MAINTAIN THE PROPER PH BALANCE IN THE BLOOD AND MAINTAIN GOOD DIGESTIVE HEALTH?

- Finding and maintaining a clean, pure water source is extremely important. I will offer a few suggestions later in the book. Our bodies need water and are made up of water. The water you consume should be as clean as possible. Adding fresh squeezed lemon or lime juice will increase the alkalinity of the water. It is important to maintain proper hydration. Can you drink half your body weight in water a day? How about making a conscious decision to just increase your water consumption? Limit your water intake right before and after a meal. This helps the digestive system process foods more effectively and efficiently.

- It is important to chew your foods very well. Your digestive system will function better if you thoroughly chew your foods before swallowing. Your body will not have to work as hard to break down the food.

- Bowel movements including their smell, shape, and color will give you clues as to how well or not well your digestive system is working. Chronic constipation and diarrhea are also good indicators that something is not functioning at its' fullest potential. Your child should have a bowel movement every day. Ideally, it will look almost banana shaped. It should not look discolored, loose, overly smelly or appear as little nuggets. Switching to a diet that promotes the proper pH balance will give the body the fiber it needs to stay regulated.

- The basic idea is to rid or minimize your daily diet of processed foods that have additives, chemicals, and preservatives. Begin or continue to increase your daily consumption of fruits, vegetables, legumes (beans), whole grains, organic and lean cuts of meat, healthy oils, healthier snack options, and fish on occasion.

- Increase the amount and different types of vegetables consumed on a daily basis. Vegetables contain vitamins, minerals, amino acids, calcium, fiber, chlorophyll, and enzymes. Raw vegetables are great. However, if you suffer from a digestive disorder slightly cooked or steamed vegetables is important for you to consider. Steaming vegetables is also a good option, as you will not lose as many nutrients as you do boiling them in water. The darker and brighter the skin, the more nutrients it contains. Homemade soups and broths are another way to receive nutrients while giving your digestive system a break from having to work so hard to break the food down.

- Reduce or eliminate sugar, white flour, fatty meats, fatty oils, fast-food, and dairy products from your daily diet. By simply reducing the junk foods, fast-foods, and convenience foods from your child's daily diet, you will significantly reduce exposure to many man-made toxins and chemicals.

- Eat 3 meals throughout the day. If you snack in between meals, make it a healthy snack. Can you start your morning off with a glass of water as you get out of bed? Limit your late night eating and try not to overeat at any one time.
- Reduce stress and get enough sleep each night.
- If you have a child that runs away from anything that resembles a vegetable, I recommend that you keep introducing them at lunch and dinner as encouragement and modeling is important. If your child just won't try them, see if they are willing to try this product: Super Greens (www.innerlightinc.com). This product is a powder and can be added to drinks. Most health food stores also carry vitamins or powders that contain the nutrients found in vegetables.
- Take nutritional supplements or vitamins. An educated practitioner is one of the best aids you can have in creating an approach or treatment plan that strives to reduce physical symptoms. Maintaining a healthy digestive balance and the proper pH balance in your blood is important for healing and health. Depending on what your body requires or suffers from, a professional can help you determine the appropriate treatment plan. I am hesitant to get specific about the types of foods that are beneficial, especially if you have been diagnosed with a disease or have chronic symptoms. The list of variables as to why you have symptoms needs to be explored. I cannot give you those answers. I do know that by following the above suggestions you will begin to create a healthier balance in your body. For example, someone that suffers from Candida should eliminate sugar as much as possible from their diet. There are certain fruits and packaged foods that are better than others. A person that has a lactose intolerance or sensitivity will need to avoid dairy products. Someone that suffers from Celiac disease has to avoid products containing gluten. All three diets will require a slightly different approach but the concept is the same. However, we could all reduce our consumption of sugar, gluten, and dairy. An important thing to consider is reducing animal products in our foods and increasing the quantity of vegetables consumed on a daily and on-going basis. Please note the vitamin and supplement industry is now big business and growing steadily. Not all products work as effectively as they are advertised. I don't want you to throw your money away on a product that is not beneficial to you or your child. Please seek assistance on which products to purchase. I have used Metagenics, Advance Naturals, Nordic Naturals, Xymogen, and Boiron (homeopathic remedies).
- As a starting point, you can refer to pages 258 to research homeopathic practitioners in your area.

- Ask family, friends, or professionals in your area for a referral to the type of nutritionist or practitioner you are seeking. There are many types of jobs and people who specialize in nutrition. I believe the important point to consider is how does your practitioner connect food to optimizing your overall health? How does your practitioner connect the toxicity of our environment to the symptoms you are reporting? An RD is a registered dietician with a four year degree. A RD typically works in an institutional type setting such as a hospital, school, government program, or nursing home. Their job is to meet the nutritional needs of the clients they serve. A Certified Clinical Nutritionist (CCN) also requires a four year degree with further education. The CCN will use supplements and other intervention therapies to obtain optimal health for you. Someone with a Certified Nutrition Specialist degree (CNS) completes an extensive education program including a master's or doctorate program. They will have also had a long internship program. There are also skilled practitioners that specialize in Chinese medicine, herbs, functional medicine, etc.
- Increase intake of probiotic food (containing healthy bacteria).

"When diet is wrong, medicine is of no use. When diet is correct, medicine is of no need."

~ ANCIENT AYURVEDIC PROVERB

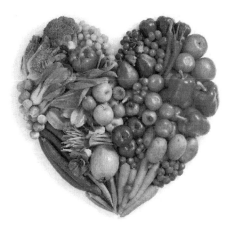

<u>Antibiotics</u>

I am not a scientist or a doctor. I cannot break down the evolution of antibiotics, their different classifications, and what they mean specifically. Nor do I think it is important to necessarily understand that information in the context of this book. I can give you in layman's terms some important points to consider when deciding if your child needs to take an antibiotic for an infection.

Everybody has taken an antibiotic or several over the course of their lifetime when they are sick or beset with symptoms. There is nothing unusual about this practice in our culture today. Some people take daily medications to help with chronic conditions such as diabetes, high blood pressure or cholesterol, heart disease, arthritis, migraines, AIDS, digestive conditions, asthma, diabetes, Lyme disease, and all types of cancers. We can also now take medications to help us with our anxiety, morning sickness, acne, sexual desires or inadequacies, behavioral and neurological disorders, and everyday colds, flu's, and viruses. Basically, we can take a pill to help with everything that is wrong or perceived to be wrong with our bodies today. It is up to each of us to make an informed decision about the benefits or risks of taking antibiotics or medications. It is not my place or position to tell you that you should or should not do something. That is for you to decide. If you take your child to the pediatrician for a sick visit, I am pretty confident your next stop will be the pharmacy to fill a prescription. I did this for years with Frankie! What I would like to share with you is what happens to our "insides" when we take an antibiotic or perhaps too many antibiotics several times a year. Antibiotics can often lead to a disruption of the normal flora and intricate balance in the digestive system.

The basic definition of antibiotic refers to a medication used to kill or deactivate bacteria in our body. It makes sense to say we take an antibiotic to kill the bacterial infection in our body when we are sick. Examples of types of illnesses caused by bacteria include: strep throat, ear infections, tuberculosis, urinary tract infections, E. coli, salmonella, typhoid, staph infections, sinus infections, bronchitis, Lyme disease, acne, gonorrhea, bacterial meningitis, and bacterial pneumonia. A viral infection is an infection that is caused by a virus. A virus requires a living host such as a person, plant, or animal. Examples of viral infections include: the common cold, chicken pox, flu, AIDS, mononucleosis, measles, mumps, rabies, hand, mouth-and-foot disease, gastroenteritis, croup, and hepatitis A, B, and C. An antibiotic will do nothing to help with a viral infection. However, these conditions may produce an increase in symptoms such as mucus. An increase in mucus can create an environment that allows bacteria to flourish, in which case an antibiotic may be helpful. I would speak with your doctor about this issue and take the antibiotic as a last resort. When we take an antibiotic for an infection, we are bypassing the immune system and its ability to defend against the "foreign" invader or invaders.

The immune system is a complex system within the body designed to defend the body from a "foreign" invader. An invader can be a bacteria, virus, parasite, mold, microbe, toxin or fungus. These invaders are usually called antigens. The body is designed to identify the antigen and destroy it. When an antigen is identified in the body, the immune system immediately responds and sends signals to cells, organs, and tissues to destroy that antigen.

Bacteria are living, single-celled organisms or microbes present in all of our bodies. They can be found in our eyes, mouth, intestines, and skin. We all have good and bad bacteria in our bodies. We rely on our digestive and immune systems to unknowingly balance the two in order to keep us physically healthy. It would make sense that we want more good bacteria than invasive, harmful bacteria.

Candida albicans is a type of yeast that is also naturally present in our digestive system. There is "good" yeast and "bad" yeast or fungus. It is completely different than bacteria and is naturally not as prevalent as bacteria in the body. The healthy balance of bacteria, acid, and yeast in our bodies is often referred to as our normal flora. This normal flora works together to sustain our digestive wellness and our wellness as a whole. The delicate balancing act of these organisms can become disrupted by antibiotics, poor diet, stress, and environmental chemicals and toxins.

Yeast is typically a non-invasive or non-threatening organism. This non-invasive, single cell form requires oxygen and battles it out with the other organisms for oxygen and space in our intestinal tract. In essence, each of our bodies has a type of checks and balance system. Yeast usually resides in small numbers in comparison to the bacteria in our bodies. They are able to survive in a dark, warm, and moist environment. The healthy body will keep the good bacteria plentiful and yeast at a minimum. A healthy digestive system will keep bacteria and yeast regulated and will help to maintain the proper pH balance.

Taking an antibiotic to ward off the illness or sickness we have been diagnosed with kills both the good and bad bacteria. It kills all the bacteria! The normal flora (acid, enzymes, yeast, and bacteria) in our digestive system is now unbalanced. What happens to our bodies when the antibiotic has wiped out both the good and bad bacteria? What happens when your child has been on several doses of an antibiotic during their lifetime? Well, that non-threatening yeast has the opportunity and potential to mutate and unknowingly become threatening to our overall health. This is when the balance of yeast in the body is interrupted and can have devastating effects on a child or adult. When the yeast in your body thrives, unchecked by the disappearance of bacteria, it will begin a mutation process that transforms the healthy yeast into an invading fungus. After one or several antibiotic treatments, the digestive system is missing the proper balance of normal flora. This changes the digestive environment and allows the yeast to begin to morph into a fungus. The interesting thing about the yeast in our bodies is that its structure changes shape as it transforms from naturally occurring yeast into a fungus. It will mutate, becoming a multiple-cellular organism.

How does the "good" yeast morph into the "bad fungus"? In the right environment, yeast will transform into a fungus that no longer thrives on oxygen. In other words, it no longer needs air to survive. The good bacteria are no longer in the digestive system and this provides the right environment for the yeast to grow. It begins to grow "spiderlike" legs as it tries to break out of the intestinal tract. It is searching, exploring, probing, and in hot pursuit of expanding. Why does the fungus want to leave the intestinal tract? What is it in search of? It is in search of food. The type of food yeast crave the most is SUGAR! The yeast is in search of the one thing that will promote its growth. Yeast do not care if the sugar is from a piece of fruit, an organic or healthier product containing sugar (an example would be a replacement for maple syrup called agave), or from a candy bar. Sugar is sugar. This is an important detail as it relates to the diets our children consume on a daily basis.

The holes made by the yeast in the intestinal tract are too small for the yeast to physically escape into other parts of the body. The waste or toxins left by the fungus leak into the blood causing symptoms throughout the entire body. These toxins once in the blood cause inflammation and allergic reactions. It is interesting to note that inflammation is being studied as the cause of asthma, headaches, irritability, heart disease, autoimmune diseases, fatigue, and more. Bodily inflammation is a huge concern for anyone suffering from physical ailments. I have read there are approximately eighty toxins the fungus produces and leaves for the body to absorb. The entire body has the potential to be damaged by the negative effects of yeast overgrowth. This is a perfect example of how our bodies can be looked at from a perspective of wholeness or oneness. A problem such as Candida starts in the digestive system. Over time, symptoms begin to include other areas of the body and its systems. These symptoms can be contributed to an unbalance in the digestive system as well as an unbalance in the acidity/alkalinity of our blood.

Suggestions for digestive balance and overall health should you or your child requires an antibiotic:

It would be beneficial to you or your child to confirm and question your doctor about whether or not your sickness or symptoms are the result of a bacterial infection or a viral infection.

IF YOU CHOOSE TO TAKE AN ANTIBIOTIC:

- Increase your intake of probiotics found in food or supplements after you have finished the antibiotic. This will help to replace the elimination of healthy bacteria in your gut after the course of treatment. You can purchase probiotic supplements that contain Lactobacillus acidophilus and Bifidobactrerium bifidum. Examples of foods containing probiotics include: yogurt, kefir, miso, unfermented sauerkraut, and kombucha (fermented tea). If you suffer from Candida, fermented foods are not recommended as they are acid forming and create mucus.
- Drink plenty of water
- Rest/sleep

WHETHER YOU CHOOSE TO TAKE AN ANTIBIOTIC OR NOT:

- Boost your immune system and allow it to do its job
- Eat more high fiber foods
- Drink plenty of water
- Sleep and nurture yourself
- Visit a health food store and purchase homeopathic remedies to help you with symptoms. You can locate a health food store in your area by going to http://www.greenpeople.org/healthfood.htm
- Allow your body to heal on its own
- Eat healthy by cutting out processed foods
- Reduce or eliminate sugar
- Taking supplements will be helpful. For example, zinc and selenium help to boost your immune system naturally
- Garlic, wasabi, cranberries, honey, onions, and some fresh herbs (cinnamon, cilantro, ginger, oregano, and parsley) contain antibacterial properties
- Drink healthy teas
- Increase vegetables and healthy food choices
- Consume homemade or organic broths and soups

COMMON SYMPTOMS/ILLNESSES/DISEASES THAT CAN BE ASSOCIATED WITH YEAST OVERGROWTH (CANDIDA):

- General "ill" feeling
- Headache
- Fatigue
- Dark circles under eyes
- Nasal congestion
- Asthma
- Sugar cravings

- Food sensitivities and allergies
- Chemical sensitivities
- Depression
- Coughing
- Wheezing
- Hyperactivity
- Learning problems
- Fatigue
- Thrush, acne, eczema, diaper and skin rashes
- Ear infections
- Sinus related illnesses
- Colic
- Irritability and moodiness
- Gas, diarrhea, constipation, and other digestive problems
- Muscle and joint pain
- Chronic colds
- Sleep problems
- Possible link to autism
- Autoimmune diseases (there are over eighty)
- Upper respiratory infections
- Poor memory and mental fogginess
- Weight gain or loss
- PMS
- Cancer
- Blood-sugar levels

If you or your child suffers from any of the above symptoms, conditions, or diseases, there is the distinct possibility that yeast overgrowth can be a contributing factor to the health issues you are facing. I have included several yeast related evaluations below. I invite you to take a few minutes and complete the tests below to find out if your physical health is being adversely affected by Candida. See for yourself!

Test #1 Are Your Health Problems Yeast Connected?

If your answer is "yes" to any question, circle the number in the right hand column. When you've completed the questionnaire, add up the points. Your score will help you determine the possibility (or probability) that your health problems are yeast related.

	YES	NO	Score
1. Have you taken repeated or prolonged courses of antibacterial drugs?	☐	☐	4
2. Have you been bothered by recurrent vaginal, prostate, or urinary-tract infections?	☐	☐	3
3. Do you feel "sick all over," yet the cause hasn't been found?	☐	☐	2
4. Are you bothered by hormone disturbances including PMS, menstrual irregularities, sexual dysfunction, sugar craving, low body temperature, or fatigue?	☐	☐	2
5. Are you unusually sensitive to tobacco smoke, perfumes, colognes, and other chemical odors?	☐	☐	2
6. Are you bothered by memory or concentration problems? Do you sometimes feel "spaced out"?	☐	☐	2

7. Have you taken prolonged courses of prednisone or other steroids; or have you taken "the pill" for more than three years? ☐ ☐ 2

8. Do some foods disagree with you or trigger your symptoms? ☐ ☐ 1

9. Do you suffer with constipation, diarrhea, bloating, or abdominal pain? ☐ ☐ 1

10. Does your skin itch, tingle, or burn; or is it unusually dry; or are you bothered by rashes? ☐ ☐ 1

Scoring for women: If your score is 9 or more, your health problems are probably yeast-connected. If your score is 12 or more, your health problems are almost certainly yeast-connected.

Scoring for men: If your score is 7 or more, your health problems are probably yeast-connected. If your score is 10 or more, your health problems are almost certainly yeast-connected.

The Candida Questionnaire is reprinted from *The Yeast Connection Handbook* by William Crook, M.D.

Test #2 Yeast Questionnaire for Children's Candida

Scoring this children's Candida questionnaire should help you and your physician evaluate the role Candida albicans contributes to your child's health problems.

1. During the two years before your child was born were you bothered by recurrent vaginitis, menstrual irregularities, premenstrual tension, fatigue, headache, depression, digestive disorders, or "feeling bad" all over? (30 points)

○ No   ○ Yes

2. Was your child bothered by Thrush (white coating on tongue or lips)? (Score 10 if mild, score 20 if severe)

○ No   ○ Mild   ○ Severe

3. Was your child bothered by frequent diaper rashes in infancy? (Score 10 if mild, score 20 if severe or persistent)

○ No   ○ Mild   ○ Severe

4. During infancy was your child bothered by colic and irritability lasting over three months? (Score 10 if mild, score 20 if moderate to severe)

○ No   ○ Mild   ○ Severe

5. Are his/her symptoms worse on damp days or in damp or moldy places? (20 points)

○ No   ○ Yes

6. Has your child been bothered by recurrent or persistent athlete's foot or chronic fungus infections on his/her skin or nails? (30 points)

○ No   ○ Yes

7. Has your child been bothered by recurrent hives, eczema, or other skin problems? (10 points)

○ No   ○ Yes

8. Has your child received:

a. Four or more courses of antibiotic drugs during the past year? Or has he or she received continuous prophylactic courses of antibiotic drugs? (60 points)

○ No   ○ Yes

b. Eight or more courses of "broad spectrum antibiotics (such as amoxicillin, Keflex, Septra, Bactrim, or Ceclor) during the past three years? (40 points)

○ No   ○ Yes

9. Has your child experienced recurrent ear problems? (20 points)

○ No   ○ Yes

10. Has your child had tubes inserted in his or her ears? (10 points)

○ No ○ Yes

11. Has your child been labeled "hyperactive? (Score 10 if mild, score 20 if moderate to severe)

○ No ○ Mild ○ Moderate to Severe

12. Is your child bothered by learning problems (even though their early development history was normal)? (10 points)

○ No ○ Yes

13. Does your child have a short attention span? (10 points)

○ No ○ Yes

14. Is your child persistently irritable, unhappy, and hard to please? (10 points)

○ No ○ Yes

15. Has your child been bothered by persistent or recurrent digestive problems including constipation, diarrhea, bloating, or excessive gas? (Score 10 if mild; score 20 if moderate; score 30 if severe)

○ No ○ Mild ○ Moderate ○ Severe

16. Has your child been bothered by persistent nasal congestion, cough, and or wheezing? (10 points)

○ No ○ Yes

17. Is your child unusually tired, unhappy, or depressed? (Score 10 if mild, score 20 if severe)

○ No ○ Mild ○ Severe

18. Has your child been bothered by recurrent headaches, abdominal pain, or muscle aches? (Score 10 if mild, score 20 if severe)

○ No ○ Mild ○ Severe

19. Does your child crave sweets? (10 points)

○ No ○ Yes

20. Does exposure to perfume, insecticides, gas, or other chemicals provoke moderate to severe symptoms? (30 points)

○ No ○ Yes

21. Does tobacco smoke really bother him or her? (20 points)

O   No   O   Yes

22. Do you feel that your child isn't well, yet diagnostic tests and studies haven't revealed the cause? (10 points)

O   No   O   Yes

Your Score is [   ] [Clear]

Score of 60 or more: Candida Yeasts possibly play a role in causing health problems in your child.

Score of 100 or more: Candida Yeasts probably play a role in causing health problems in your child.

Score of 140 or more: Candida Yeasts almost certainly play a role in causing health problems in your child.

The Candida Questionnaire is reprinted from *The Yeast Connection Handbook* by William Crook, M.D.

Test #3 Check list for Candida albicans

This test reviews the signs and symptoms to determine if you have Candida albicans yeast infection overgrowth.

Candida albicans yeast infection overgrowth or Candida Overgrowth (CO) symptoms are so numerous and seemingly unrelated that they can be confusing to both doctor and patient. The majority of people who have CO do not realize they have it until they become seriously ill. Why? Because CO not only steals nutrients from the food you eat, it then poisons the tissues with waste material containing over eighty toxins. Candida albicans is linked, directly or indirectly, to the following list of conditions and symptoms. A "symptom" is an outward sign that points to a deeper problem.

Review the eighty likely symptoms listed below to see if any apply to you. Give yourself one point for each of those which you have had persistently (for a month or longer and either currently, or at any time in the past).

Digestive Troubles

- Bad Breath
- Gas/Bloating
- Indigestion
- Diarrhea
- Constipation
- Intestinal Pain
- Low Blood Sugar
- Food / Sugar Cravings
- Mouth or Stomach Ulcers
- Allergies (Air or Food)
- Food Sensitivities
- Heartburn
- Dry Mouth
- Receding Gums
- Hemorrhoids, Rectal Itch
- Irritable Bowel

Behavioral

- Antisocial Behavior
- Suicidal Tendencies
- Insomnia
- Depression
- Anxiety, High-Strung Personality
- Irritability

Skin & Joint Problems

- Thrush, Diaper Rash
- Acne, Skin Rash, or Hives
- Dry Skin and Itching
- Finger, Toe, or Foot Fungus
- Athlete's Foot
- Liver Spots
- Water Retention
- Joint Pain
- Muscle Aches
- Numbness

Troubles

- Hyperactivity
- Attention Deficit Disorder
- Lack of Impulse Control'

Female Problems

- Infertility
- Vaginal Yeast Infection
- Menstrual Problems
- PMS Symptoms
- Bladder Infections
- Endometriosis
- No Sex Drive
- Hormonal Imbalance
- Iron Deficiency

Mental & Emotional

- Dizziness
- Mental Fogginess (Confused, spaced-out, blank stares, daydreaming)
- Inability to Concentrate (having to reread the same thing twice)
- Poor memory (where are my car keys or why did I come into this room?)
- Mood Swings
- Headaches

Immune Problems

- Lethargy/Laziness
- Chronic Fatigue
- Asthma, Hay Fever
- Colds & Flu
- Puffy Eyes

- Respiratory Problems
- Chemical Sensitivity
- Epstein Barr Virus
- Adrenal/Thyroid Failure
- Cold/Shaky
- Ear Infections
- Chronic sore throat
- Post nasal drip
- Hair Loss
- Stuffed Sinus (Sinusitis)
- Being Overweight
- Being Underweight
- Diabetes
- Burning Eyes
- Premature Aging
- Autism

YOUR ADDED SCORE IS _____ (one point per symptom)

0-4 points - Indicates variations of normal living (unless persistent and severe).

5-9 Points - Indicates a Clear Pattern that shows likely development of CO Dysbiosis.

10 or more - Indicates Strong Pattern and almost certain CO Dysbiosis.

The Candida Questionnaire is reprinted from *The Yeast Connection Handbook* by William Crook, M.D.

Test #4 CANDIDA QUESTIONNAIRE AND SCORE SHEET

This questionnaire is designed for adults and the scoring system isn't appropriate for children. It lists factors in your medical history which promote the growth of the common yeast Candida albicans (Section A) and symptoms commonly found in individuals with yeast-connected illness (Sections B and C).

For each "Yes" answer in Section A, circle the "Point Score" in that section. Total your score and record it in the box at the end of the section. Then move on to Sections B and C and score as directed.

Answering and scoring this questionnaire will help you and your physician evaluate the possible role of yeast overgrowth in contributing to your health problems. Yet, it will not provide an automatic yes or no answer.

SECTION A: HISTORY

Point

Score

1. Have you taken tetracycline's (Sumy in®, Kanamycin®, Vibramycin®, Minocen®, etc.) or other antibiotics for acne for one month (or longer)? 35 points

2. Have you at any time in your life taken other broad-spectrum antibiotics for respiratory, urinary, or other infections (for two months or longer or in shorter courses four or more times in a one-year period)? 35 points

3. Have you taken a broad-spectrum antibiotic drug, even a single course? 6 points

4. Have you at any time in your life been bothered by persistent prostatitis, vaginitis, or other problems affecting your reproductive organs? 25 points

5. Have you been pregnant two or more times? 5 points

   Have you been pregnant one time? 3 points

6. Have you taken birth control pills for more than two years? 15 points

   For 6 months to two years? 8 points

7. Have you taken prednisone, Decadron®, or other cortisone-type drugs?

   For more than two weeks? 15 points

   For two weeks or less? 6 points

8. Does exposure to perfumes, insecticides, fabric shop odors, or other chemicals provoke moderate to severe symptoms? 20 points

   Mild symptoms? 5 points

9. Are your symptoms worse on damp, muggy days, or in moldy places? 20 points

10. Have you had athlete's foot, ring worm, jock itch, or other chronic fungus infections of the skin or nails? Have such infections been

    Severe or persistent? 20 points

    Mild to moderate? 10 points

11. Do you crave sugar? 10 points

12. Do you crave breads? 10 points

13. Do you crave alcoholic beverages? 10 points

14. Does tobacco smoke *really* bother you? 10 points

Total Score, Section A _____

SECTION B: MAJOR SYMPTOMS

For each symptom which is present, enter the appropriate score to the right of each symptom:

If a symptom is **occasional or mild** . . . . score 3 points.

If a symptom is **frequent and/or moderately severe** . . . . score 6 points.

If a symptom is **severe and/or disabling** . . . . .score 9 points.

Add total score for this section and record it in the box at the end of this section.

Point
Score

1. Fatigue or lethargy
2. Feeling of being drained
3. Poor memory
4. Feeling spacey or unreal
5. Inability to make decisions
6. Numbness, burning, or tingling

7. Insomnia

8. Muscle aches

9. Muscle weakness or paralysis

10. Pain or swelling in joints

11. Abdominal pain

12. Constipation

13. Diarrhea

14. Bloating, belching, or intestinal gas

15. Troublesome vaginal burning, itching, or discharge

16. Prostatitis

17. Impotence

18. Loss of sexual desire or feeling

19. Endometriosis or infertility

20. Cramps or other menstrual irregularities

21. Premenstrual tension

22. Attacks of anxiety or crying

23. Cold hands or feet and/or chilliness

24. Shaking or irritable when hungry

Total Score, Section B _____

(While the symptoms in this section occur commonly in patients with yeast connected illness, they also occur commonly in patients who do not have Candida.)

SECTION C: OTHER SYMPTOMS

For each symptom which is present, enter the appropriate score to the right of the symptom:

If a symptom is **occasional or mild** . . . . .score 1 point.

If a symptom is **frequent and/or moderately severe** . . . . .score 2 points.

If a symptom is **severe and/or persistent** . . . . .score 3 points.

Add total score for this section and record it in the box at the end of this section.

Point

Score

1. Drowsiness
2. Irritability or jitteriness
3. Lack of coordination
4. Inability to concentrate
5. Frequent mood swings
6. Headache
7. Dizziness or loss of balance
8. Pressure above ear or feeling of head swelling
9. Tendency to bruise easily
10. Chronic rashes or itching
11. Psoriasis or recurrent hives
12. Indigestion or heartburn
13. Food sensitivity or intolerance
14. Mucus in stools
15. Rectal itching
16. Dry mouth or throat
17. Rash or blisters in mouth
18. Bad breath
19. Foot, hair, or body odor not relieved by washing
20. Nasal congestion or post nasal drip
21. Nasal itching
22. Sore throat
23. Laryngitis, loss of voice
24. Cough or recurrent bronchitis
25. Pain or tightness in chest
26. Wheezing or shortness of breath
27. Urinary frequency, urgency, or incontinence
28. Burning on urination
29. Spots in front of eyes or erratic vision

30. Burning or tearing of eyes

31. Recurrent infections or fluid in ears

32. Ear pain or deafness

Total Score, Section C:

Total Score, Section B:

Total Score, Section A:

GRAND TOTAL SCORE (Add up Total Score from Sections A, B, and C):

Scores in women will run higher as seven items in the questionnaire apply exclusively to women, while only two apply exclusively to men.

Yeast-connected health problems are almost certainly present in women with scores more than 180, and in men with scores more than 140.

Yeast-connected health problems are probably present in women with scores more than 120, and in men with scores more than 90.

Yeast-connected health problems are possibly present in women with scores more than 60, and in men with scores more than 40.

With scores of less than 60 in women and 40 in men, yeasts are less apt to cause health problems.

The Candida Questionnaire is reprinted from *The Yeast Connection Handbook* by William Crook, M.D.

If you seek a different path in regard to maintaining your health or the health of your child, understanding the ways in which your digestive system functions is important. By changing your diet and collaborating with a knowledgeable practitioner, you can begin to eliminate your symptoms, possibly (and probably) reduce medications and antibiotics, educate yourself on your body, become empowered, take control, and feel better.

Another way that we can improve and enhance the functioning of our children's bodies is by better understanding their external environment. This includes the toxins and chemicals that have the potential to cause immediate and long-term consequences to their health.

Resources for Candida albicans and overall digestive health:

1. *Yeast Connection Handbook* by William G. Crook, M.D.
2. *Complete Candida Yeast Guidebook* by Jeanne Marie Martin
3. *The Candida Cure* by Ann Boroch
4. www.candidasupport.org
5. www.nationalcandidacenter.com
6. National Association of Nutrition Professionals (NANP) http://www.nanp.org
7. American Holistic Medical Association (AHMA) http:www.holisticmedicine.org
8. *pH Miracle* by Robert O. Young & Shelley Redford Young. This book will provide invaluable information and insight while providing an extensive list of foods to eat and foods to avoid. The authors explain in detail the connection to our health problems as it relates to Alkaline vs. Acid (pH balance).
9. http://www.youtube.com/watch?v=DdjLHlltiUE. This is a link to a You Tube video that explores the connection between acid/alkalinity and our overall health. It explores the pH balance.
10. *Digestive Wellness* by Elizabeth Lipski

References

1. William G Crook, M.D. The Yeast Connection Handbook. Square One Publisher, 1996, 1997, 1999 and 2000.

2. National Candida Center, "What Causes Candida", Accessed April 26, 2014, http;//www. nationalcandidacenter.com/candida-causes/

3. National Candida Center, "What is candida Yeast infection", Accessed April 26, 2014, http:// www.nationalcandidacenter.com/candida-what/

4. Don't Die Early, "pH Definition, Accessed July 23, 2011, http://www.dontdieearly.com/ ph-level/ph-definition.htm

5. What is a Viral Infection, "Viral infection: Definition", Accessed September 9, 2012, http:// www.coldflu.about.com/od/glossary/g/viralinfection.htm

6. Bacterial vs. Viral Infections: Causes and Treatments, "Bacterial and Viral Infections", Accessed October 24, 2012, http://www.webmd.com/a-to-z-guides/bacterial-and-viral-infections

7. National Candida Center, "NCC: pH Miracle, New Biology, Alkalization.wmv", Accessed August 12, 2012, http://www.youtube.com/watch?v=DdjLHlltiUE

Section 2
The Chemical Problem Today in a Nutshell: The Poisoning of Our Children

The chapters in this section of the book will help identify the main sources of chemicals and toxins in your child's environment. Your child does not need to be sick or have chronic symptoms to eliminate chemicals, processed foods, and antibiotics from their daily lives. It is important to eliminate these toxins in an effort to make his or her environment safe and their bodies strong enough to fight the diseases that are eventually and unfortunately headed their way. Actually, it does not have to be this way. We do not need to expect to develop cancer, major digestive disorders, diabetes, heart disease, high blood pressure, Candida, high cholesterol, etc. in this lifetime. We can begin to reduce our exposure to chemicals by choosing to eat foods that are alive and provide our body with the proper nutrients. The food industry, the medical profession, corporations, the pharmaceutical companies, and our own government are not going to do this job as thoroughly or as adequately as you. They just aren't, plain and simple.

THE MAIN SOURCES OF TOXINS AND CHEMICALS THAT WILL BE EXPLORED IN THIS SECTION OF THE BOOK INCLUDE:

- Food/Factory Farming
- Cleaning Supplies/Household Items
- Daily Beauty Products
- Water

It is my hope that the chapters you are about to read are easy to understand and begin to make sense on a basic or general level. I have tried my best to break the following information into ideas that are simplistic in nature and easy to read. There is so much information coming from a myriad of perspectives and experts. This means navigating your way through the intricate and confusing maze of the food industry can be a daunting and difficult challenge. If you decide that making changes to your child's or family's daily environment is important, please note that the change you are seeking will not happen overnight. Continue to work on it day by day.

We live in a world that has been made simple. Everything we need or desire is a step away and within easy reach. We now have the ability to access information in seconds, purchase prepackaged foods and meals for our convenience, and shop anytime and anywhere. I am not saying this is necessarily a bad thing. However, in its commercialized simplicity, we have created a toxic environment for our children on a physical and emotional level.

So what can "everyday" parents do to ensure their child's environment is free from as many chemicals and toxins as possible? I invite you to challenge yourself to think outside the box about what is considered "normal" in our culture today. Reducing the chemicals our children are exposed to in medications, foods, cleaning supplies, water, or other environmental pollutants is something all parents should be aware of and concerned about. As I know you are! Where do we begin making such a transformation you might ask? Educating ourselves is the first step. Let us begin by looking at some of the challenges our children face today.

CHAPTER 6
The Next Generation

"The world is a dangerous place, not because of those who do evil, but because of those who look on and do nothing."
-ALBERT EINSTEIN

Why does it seem so hard being a parent in today's world? It seems more complicated for us now than it was for our parents. Maybe that is a relative statement and each generation of parents feels the same way. Today we are facing an epidemic of childhood obesity and an alarming increase of children with asthma, environmental allergies, autism, ADHD, ADD, learning disabilities, diabetes, food allergies, behavioral problems, digestive disorders, mental health issues, increased levels of stress, and more. Since I have become more aware of food and our environment, I am finding more and more articles, websites, television show segments, books, and having more conversations with family and friends that revolve around these issues.

Below are titles of a small group of newspaper and web articles I have found in the last few years to highlight my point. The titles alone signify that something is wrong.

RECENT ARTICLE HEADLINES

- Asthma Rates Rising, but Cause Unclear
- Some Chicken May Contain Arsenic, FDA Says
- Pesticide Exposure in Womb Affects I.Q.
- Is Sugar Toxic?
- Editorial: Hiding the Truth about Factory Farms
- More Tainted Foods Coming From China?
- Kids are Not as Healthy as Parents Think
- Doctors Seek Better Regulation of Toxins
- Combat Chronic Illness in Children with Preventative Care
- Energy Drinks Hot, Medical Jitters are Hotter
- Roundup Birth Defects: Regulators Knew World's Best-Selling Herbicide Causes Problems, New Report Finds
- Latest Toxic Toy Recall: Lead and Cadmium in Toys and Jewelry
- Painkillers, Antibiotics, Growth Hormones Among The 20 Chemicals Found in Typical Glass of Milk
- Mice Study Finds Air Pollution Linked to Depression, Memory Issues
- Is Your Food as Healthy as You Think?
- Sugar Sweetened Drinks Linked With High Blood Pressure
- Think Dirty App Reveals Just How Toxic Certain Beauty Products Are
- Measles Cases at Highest Level in Nearly 20 Years, CDC Reports
- High-Fat Diets Linked to Some Types of Breast Cancer
- 1 in 13 Children Taking Psychiatric Medication in U.S.
- Glyphosate Found at High Levels in Mothers' Breast Milk

It is becoming more and more apparent to me that companies are determining the success of a product based on the financial profit and not on the quality of that specific product. I understand the concept of our capitalistic society, along with the dynamics of supply and demand. However, in the long run we are hurting each other. Our government, who has determined that they must regulate just about every aspect of our lives, is failing to protect us. I would also hesitantly say that we are allowing companies and the government to control our lives. Generally speaking, it is no longer about us. It is not about the citizens, your children, or the everyday consumer. Politics has entered the food, pharmaceutical, and medical industries. I am not naïve enough to assume that this happen overnight. I will suggest that we are at a major turning point in this country regarding just about most freedoms that this country was founded upon. This absolutely includes our government regulated oversight into the national food supply. This is a very scary and real concern for us, our children, and future generations. We must begin to take control of our lives and not stay dependent on other people, companies, or institutions to dictate how we live our lives.

The Health of Our Children
Basic Facts

According to America's Children in Brief: Key National indicators of Well-being: in 2011 there were 73.9 million children in the United States. They represented 24 percent of the entire U.S. population. By 2050, that number will increase to 101.6 million children. In 2010, 22 percent or 16.4 million children lived in poverty. Of those, 44 percent were living in food insecure households meaning they lacked consistent access to adequate food. According to this study, health care is defined as the prevention, treatment, and maintenance of illness as well as the promotion of emotion, behavioral, and physical well-being. In 2010, 7.3 million children had no healthcare coverage.

We have all heard the phrase that children are the future. They are the future entrepreneurs, doctors, teachers, scientists, nurses, business executives, craftsman, architects, musicians, small business owners, parents, engineers, service workers, and so much more. Unfortunately, this generation of children is facing huge obstacles in terms of their overall health (physical, emotional, and environmental). These obstacles will directly impact their lives and the lives of those around them at some point in their future.

Below are some statistics on common diseases and conditions that are posing significant health problems for children today.

Asthma is a chronic disease in which the airways become blocked or narrowed. Symptoms include difficulty breathing, wheezing, coughing, and tightness in the chest.

Statistics:

- 20 million Americans suffer from asthma (one in fifteen Americans).
- Nearly 7.1 million asthma sufferers are under the age of eighteen.
- Asthma is the most common chronic childhood disease affecting more than one in twenty children.
- Nearly half (44 percent) of all asthma hospitalizations are for children.
- It is the third ranking cause of hospitalizations for children.
- Asthma is the number one cause of school absenteeism among children and accounts for more than 14 million total missed days of school each year.
- The death rate for children under nineteen years old has increased by nearly 80 percent since 1980.

Attention Deficit Hyperactivity Disorder is a neurological disorder. It is characterized by developmentally inappropriate impulsivity, inattention, and in some cases hyperactivity.

Statistics:

- As of 2011, 6.4 million children (11% of children) between the ages of 4-17 have been diagnosed with ADHD. The rate of diagnosis for children has increased 3% each year from 1997-2006.
- In 2010, The CDC reported 10 percent of the children in the United States have been diagnosed with ADHD. This is an increase of almost 25 percent in four years.
- Between 2003 and 2007, one million children were given the diagnosis for the first time.
- Two-thirds of all children diagnosed with ADHD are being treated with drugs to help control symptoms.

- Since 2007, the FDA has mandated to the drug companies they make available a patient medication guide outlining the associated risks with the medications used to treat ADHD. Some of these medications can cause an increase in heart problems and psychiatric problems as well. One specific medication (Strattera) carries a different warning label. Besides the typical side effects associated with this prescribed medication, it also carries a warning of increased suicidal thoughts. My own warning statement reads: your child may kill themselves due to the side effects of this ADHD medication, but at least they won't be hyper anymore. What are we doing and by "we" I mean the scientists, doctors, and pharmaceutical companies? These companies are prescribing and selling these drugs to parents who are distressed about their child's behavior. They are concerned adults doing the very best they can to help their child. Is this really a long-term and viable option? How about yoga or meditation practices (learning to quiet the mind), natural remedies and vitamins, a decrease in sugar consumption, a vegetable dense diet, behavior modification programs, acupuncture, teaching your child how to relax, technology time-outs, etc.? Can we teach our children how to understand and manage their symptoms through the options above while using medication as a last resort and not vice versa?

Autism is a general term used to describe a group of complex developmental brain disorders. It is characterized by impaired social interaction and communication and by restricted and repetitive behavior.

Statistics:
- In the United States 1 in 68 boys and 1 in 189 girls will be diagnosed as having an Autism Spectrum Disorder this year.
- This represents a 57 percent increase from 2002–2006.
- The above statistic also represents a 600 percent increase in the number of children diagnosed with Autism in the past twenty years.
- Autism is now more common than childhood cancer, juvenile diabetes, and pediatric AIDS combined.
- Government statistics suggest the prevalence rate of autism is increasing ten to seventeen percent annually.

Diabetes is a group of diseases characterized by high blood glucose levels that result from defects in the body's ability to produce and use insulin.

Statistics:

- 25.8 million Children and adults in the United States (8.3 percent of the entire population) have diabetes.
- About 1 in every 400 children and adolescents has diabetes.
- In 2010, 1.9 million new cases of diabetes in people aged twenty and older were diagnosed.
- In 2012, the total cost (direct medical costs and reduced productivity) was $245 billion dollars.

Obesity is the result of a caloric imbalance and has both immediate and long-term health impacts.

Statistics:

- Childhood obesity has more than doubled in children and quadrupled in adolescents in the past thirty years.
- The prevalence of obesity among children from age six to eleven increased from 7 percent in 1980 to 18 percent in 2012.
- The prevalence of obesity among adolescents from ages twelve to nineteen increased from 7 percent to 18 percent.
- Obesity is also linked to a higher risk factor for heart disease, type 2 diabetes, stroke, and cancers.
- One of the most concerning statistics of childhood obesity is studies show that nearly 30 percent of the entire child population is obese. This number is projected to continue to climb.

Food Allergies are potentially serious immune responses from eating specific foods or food additives.

Statistics:

- In 2007, approximately 3 million children under the age of eighteen were reported to have a food or digestive allergy in the previous year.

- The prevalence of a food allergy among children under the age of eighteen increased 18 percent from 1997–2007.
- Food allergies affect about 6 percent of children under the age of three.
- Milk allergy is the most common childhood food allergy affecting 2.5 percent of children under the age of three.
- Peanut allergies doubled in children from 1997-2002.
- Between 150 and 200 individuals die from food allergies each year.
- 4 out of every 100 children have a food allergy.

Breast Cancer: As I was finishing up my research on childhood diseases, my younger and only sister, Rosie, discovered a lump on her breast. At the age of thirty-seven she was diagnosed with a non-genetic but invasive form of breast cancer. I am confident that anyone reading this has a family member, friend, or acquaintance battling this dreaded disease. I am including statistics on breast cancer for all the women who are reading this book.

Statistics:
- Breast cancer is the second most common cancer among American women after skin cancer. Cancer, in general, is the second leading cause of death in this country following heart disease.
- 1 out of every 8 women will develop invasive breast cancer in their lifetime. To put it a different way, 12 percent of the women in this country will be directly affected by this disease.
- There are over 2.5 million breast cancer survivors in the United States alone.

It is a remarkable testament to the millions of women who have fought the courageous fight against breast cancer or any cancer for that matter. But the question remains, why are so many women getting it in the first place? We have the medicine, machines, tests, and doctors to help treat a woman after she has been diagnosed with breast cancer, but where is the education on preventative care from the medical community?

We should all begin or continue to complete regular self-breast exams. Is it possible there is a link between breast cancer and birth control pills, hormone replacement therapy, the foods we eat, a lack of proper nutrition, and the toxicity that we now live in? As my sister began this battle, one of the first things she was instructed to do was to throw away her deodorant because it contains aluminum. Really, what guidance is that? Yes, we should all use aluminum free deodorant, but why is the general public not being informed prior to diagnosis? Why isn't it a universal teaching to educate teenage boys and girls not to use the typical deodorants that are full of chemicals including aluminum? Aluminum increases the risk of seizures, breast cancer, and Alzheimer Disease. I would think that piece of information would be given to an individual at the time of their yearly exam, sick or healthy. They also told my sister to reduce the amount of beauty products and make-up she uses on a daily basis. My guess would be because of all the chemicals found in both. Why are we waiting until someone is sick to begin educating them on some of these important issues? Can't we do better than this?

We can raise all the money in the world through fundraising efforts to research, educate, and evaluate the best treatment options for most physical diseases today. We can wear the shirts, hats, and wrist bands that bring awareness to a specific disease or place a decal on the back of the car to highlight something that is important to us. But yet I ask again, who is educating us on prevention rather than ways to control and maintain disease? Who is teaching the broader population that proper nutrition and a reduction to chemical exposure is effective in reducing the physical symptoms associated with most, if not all, of the diseases mentioned above? Who is telling you that your daily environment is toxic to your health? Who is conducting all of the research on the effectiveness of the drugs we take to fight these conditions? Who controls all of the money we unselfishly give to organizations and causes that are near and dear to our hearts? Where does all of that money go?

Do we really think the pharmaceutical giants want a cure for cancer or any other major disease for that matter? Do these giants want us to become educated and self-empowered? In my opinion, the sad truth is a resounding no. Why? Well, the answer is somewhat simplistic. They would go out of business, there would be job loss, the economy would suffer, and people would actually begin to have control over their lives. Individuals would be less dependent on a medical system and a pharmaceutical industry that is flawed. The question is: are we willing to take the time to educate ourselves and pass our knowledge onto our children and future generations?

I recently had the pleasure to listen to a speaker discuss her health journey to date at a conference in New York City. She suffers from a stage four and rare form of cancer. Thirteen years ago she decided not to pursue the typical medical route of fighting cancer (radiation, surgeries, chemotherapy, etc.) and instead changed her thought process about food. She has used this to promote healing on many different levels. She is not cancer free, but is choosing to live a life full of freedom, abundance, and choice. She is doing it with an attitude of hope that is contagious! She explains her process and the ways she transformed her kitchen to enhance her physical well-being. She writes exactly what I am trying to convey in this book. If you are reading this book, it is not working for you, and you want to get more information or a different perspective, please look her up. Her name is Kris Carr. Her best-selling books are full of energy, humor, and tons of valuable information. By the way, you do not have to have been diagnosed with cancer to learn something from her. There are resources, tons of information on healthy living, and recipes for all of us! Her books also explore the connection between the proper pH balance and our overall health.

1. <u>Crazy Sexy Cancer Survivor: More Rebellion and Fire for Your Healing</u>
2. <u>Crazy Sexy Cancer Tips</u>
3. <u>Crazy Sexy Kitchen: 150 Plant-Empowered Recipes to Ignite a Mouthwatering Revolution</u>
4. <u>Crazy Sexy Diet: Eat Your Vegies, Ignite Your Spark, and Live Like You Mean It!</u>
5. www.kriscarr.com
6. You can also YouTube her to watch her videos and interviews.

Another growing and unrelated concern in regard to our children's health is the mandatory protocol of childhood immunizations.

Childhood immunization History:

There has been much discussion in the last couple of decades in regard to the safety of vs. the need for childhood immunizations. There are two distinct and pro-foundly different schools of thought on this issue. I vaccinated all of my children without understanding the potential problems associated with this preventative measure. I did what I was told to do with limited questioning. Now that I am educating myself on the facts, I am much more aware of and concerned about the possible side effects vaccinations have on all of our children. My concern is about the ingredients and chemicals added to the vaccines.

One side of the vaccination argument is represented by the government, the pharmaceutical companies who make the vaccines, the medical community who dispenses the vaccines to the general public, and the scientific community at large. These advocates of vaccinations produce, distribute, mandate, regulate, and profit from the inoculation of our children against certain diseases. The Center for Disease Control (CDC) states an immunization is the process by which a person or animal becomes protected against a disease. This term is often used interchangeably with vaccination and vaccine. Vaccination is an injection of a dead or weakened infectious organism in order to prevent the disease it normally causes. Vaccines produce immunity and therefore protect the body from the disease. Vaccines may be administered through needle injections, by mouth, and by an aerosol spray. I also use immunization, vaccination, and vaccine interchangeably.

I believe it is fair to say that immunizations have greatly reduced or eradicated the spread of different types of infectious diseases all around the world. Millions of doses of vaccines are administered each year to children in this country and around the world. The thought is that by getting your child immunized, you contribute to the fight against and prevention of a specific disease by protecting your own child against it. You will also protect other children by making sure that your own children are healthy to be around. This side of the argument states that although there is always the potential for side effects, they are rare and do not outweigh the risks of not being vaccinated. This side also suggests that the amount of chemicals, antibiotics, preservatives, and animal by-products that are used in immunizations is minute and pose limited health risks to the recipient. We are told these ingredients are added to the vaccines for several reasons including: sterilization, to enhance the immune response, to reduce bacterial contamination, to stabilize vaccines from adverse conditions such as freezing, to provide nutrition to the cells, and to deactivate viruses in our bodies so they do not cause disease. The Center for Disease Control (CDC) also states there are rigorous policies in place to ensure safety and they maintain that immunizations are the best defense we have against infectious disease. However, the CDC also states that no vaccine is 100 percent safe or effective. What is the potential harm to our children if no vaccine is 100 percent safe?

The other side of the Vaccination argument has a very different perspective on the potential problems associated with vaccinations that are mandated by law to protect our children. This position states:

- Vaccines are not a choice. They are mandated by law. Does the government have the right to make us inject our children with foreign substances that go directly into their bloodstreams?
- Vaccines contain additives that have the potential to cause physical harm including death.
- There are known and documented side effects ranging from mild to severe.
- The side effects as a result of a vaccine are underreported. The information provided by the pharmaceutical companies and our government is skewed and does not accurately portray the actual side effects associated with these vaccines.
- There is a lack of quality information given to us by the government and pharmaceutical companies in regard to immunization safety.
- The pharmaceutical companies are the same companies conducting and compiling the research on the safety and effectiveness of these vaccines. (It is just my opinion but this seems to be a conflict of interest).

LIST OF DISEASES WE ARE PROTECTING AGAINST TODAY WHEN WE IMMUNIZE OUR CHILDREN INCLUDE:

- Diphtheria (Bacterial infection that affects the lungs)
- Hepatitis A (Infection in the liver)
- Hepatitis B (Infection in the liver)
- Human Papillomavirus (Major cause of cervical cancer and genital warts)
- Influenza (Flu)
- Measles
- Meningococcal Disease (Meningitis)
- Mumps
- Pertussis (whooping cough)
- Pneumococcal Disease (Pneumonia)
- Polio (paralysis)
- Rubella
- Tetanus
- Varicella (Chicken Pox)

SOME OF THE SIDE EFFECTS TO THESE VACCINES THAT ARE LISTED ON THE CENTER FOR DISEASE CONTROL WEBSITE INCLUDE BUT ARE NOT LIMITED TO:

- Redness/soreness at injection site
- Joint pain/muscle ache
- Headache
- Diarrhea/nausea
- Chills/fever (low/high grade)
- Cough/pneumonia
- Itching/rash
- Fatigue
- Loss of appetite
- Nasal congestion
- Allergic reaction (mild/severe)
- Seizure
- Coma
- Fainting
- Deafness
- Temporary low platelet count which can cause a bleeding disorder

One of the major concerns in the immunization controversy is the additional inclusion of heavy metals and chemicals used in the production and manufacturing of immunizations. There is a significant and growing divide in public opinion concerning the potential harm that can adversely affect our children's health as a direct result of vaccines.

Below is a list of common ingredients found in vaccines that are administered to our children today. Some of the additives added to vaccines include:

- Formaldehyde
- Thimerosal (mercury)
- Aluminum Hydroxide and Phosphate
- Aspartame

- Ammonium Sulfate
- Benzethonium Sulfate
- Beta-Propiolactone (chick embryonic fluid)
- Formalin
- Glycerin
- Monosodium L-glutamate (MSG)
- Phenol and Phenol Red
- Polydimethylsiloxane (also known as silicone)
- Soy protein
- Yeast
- Sodium Phosphate and Sodium Bicarbonate
- Potassium Chloride, Diphosphate, Glutamate, Monophosphate, Phosphate Diabasic, and Monophosphate Mombasic
- Certain antibiotics including Neomycin, Polymyxin B, Streptomycin, and Gentamicin.
- Certain vaccines contain fetal calf/bovine serum, chick embryonic fluid, and human diploid cells.

Due to the public's growing concern of vaccine safety, Congress passed the National Childhood Vaccine Injury Act in 1986. As a result of this act, the National Vaccine Injury Compensation Program was created in 1988. This program compensates individuals who have been injured by vaccines on a "no-fault" basis. "No-fault" means people filing claims are not required to prove negligence on the part of either the health care provider or the manufacturer to receive compensation. Compensation is awarded based on the Vaccine Injury Table which summarizes the adverse events caused by vaccines. This program is funded through a $ 0.75 excise tax on each vaccine your child receives. The consumer is required to pay a tax into a fund controlled by the Department of Treasury. This fund compensates other injured consumers. Since 1989, approximately 13,797 claims have been filed citing direct injury from vaccines. Of those, 3,645 claims have received monetary compensation. Another 9,786 claims have been dismissed. More than 4,509 claims are awaiting a decision by the U.S Court of Federal Claims. Most of the remaining claims have been filed as an attempt to connect autism injuries with immunizations. More than $2,700,000,000 (2.7 billion dollars) has been spent compensating individuals for their vaccination injuries. $113.2 million dollars has been paid to cover attorney's fees and other legal costs.

VAERS (Vaccine Adverse Event Reporting System) is a federal program that has been set up to track reported cases of injuries or illnesses that occur after a vaccine is given. Anyone can report a side effect. A documented report does not prove that a vaccine caused the adverse symptom(s). It only confirms that a report was filed detailing the symptom(s) after a vaccine was administered. These reports are open to the public for review. The one major problem with this system is that it is considered "passive" reporting. This means that reports are not collected by an identified agency, but only by the people who make a report. I found myself rereading a bullet point at the top of the VAERS homepage. It reads:

More than 10 million vaccines are given per year to children less than one year old and usually between two and six months of age. At this age infants are at greatest risk for certain adverse events including high fevers, seizures, and sudden infant death (SIDS). Some infants will experience these medical events shortly after a vaccination by *coincidence.*

I have one question. If I believe the above statement to be true and that vaccines cause limited side effects, why put the disclaimer at the top of page to begin with? OK, I have another question. If infants are at greater risk for possible fevers, seizures, and SIDS simply because of their age, why are we inundating their bodies with vaccines that contain live viruses, toxins, and foreign substances? It makes more sense to me to spread the vaccines out over a longer period of time and not to administer so many doses during one visit.

I took a brief look at some of the reports that were being filed by individuals, parents, and health-care practitioners following a vaccine. Below are the following symptoms I found reported on page 1 of a 33 page report:

- Muscle spasms, swelling, soreness, rash, hives, sore throat, hoarseness, fatigue, and fever.
- Headaches, shingles, chicken pox, measles, chills, wheezing, inconsolable crying, diarrhea, and bloodshot eyes.

- Neuropathy, chest pressure, vertigo, slurred speech, bloody nose, irritability, and vomiting.
- Autism, developmental regression, loss of consciousness, and seizure.
- Hospitalization, decreased language, anaphylactic reaction, Guillain-Barre Syndrome, abdominal distension, limpness, and on and on.

There is no federal agency that has publicly connected immunizations with the development or onset of autism. There are certainly a number of advocacy groups who say just the opposite. In an article published on May 11, 2011, a report was presented by safeminds.org. This study contended that the National Vaccine Injury Compensation Program has quietly compensated eighty three families involving autism out of 1300 cases of vaccine injury that resulted in childhood brain injuries. A major concern is the use of the preservative Thimerosal (mercury) in vaccines. Mercury is a heavy metal and is toxic to humans.

Both sides of the vaccination argument have their points of view, clinical research, and data to back up their particular perspectives. If childhood vaccines and their side effects for your child are a concern, there is plenty of information to help you in your decision making process. The only question I ask you is this: Is it possible that vaccines, including all of the chemical ingredients in them and the large number of vaccines administered at one time and at such a young age, are adversely affecting the very children they are intended to help? Is it possible to demand vaccines for our children that are free or reduced from chemicals, preservatives, and heavy metals? I believe that if all parents had the information from both sides of this debate, we might see a dramatic change in how vaccines are administered. I am also willing to say that less and less parents would vaccinate their children. The government, on the other hand, feels differently. The government has the ability and power to require you to take the necessary steps to vaccinate your children. According to the National Vaccine Information Center, there are specific exemptions from being required to receive vaccinations. A medical, religious, or philosophical exemption is available depending on which state you reside. I do not know how difficult it is to become exempt but, if you have questions, a good starting point or resource would be to call the National Vaccine Information Center at 1-703-938-0342 or the National Conference of State Legislatures at 1-202-624-5400.

Below is a timeline or history of immunizations and how they have evolved over the years in this country.

1940's - The mass production of vaccinations began.
* Smallpox
* DPT (Diphtheria, Tetanus, and Pertussis) (This is three different vaccines combined into one.)

A child was vaccinated at this time against four separate diseases.

1950's - Another vaccine was introduced into the immunization schedule.
* Smallpox
* DPT (Diphtheria, Tetanus, and Pertussis)
* IPV (Polio)

A child was vaccinated against five different diseases.

1960's - Three more vaccines were added to the list and combined into one vaccine called MMR.
* Smallpox
* DPT (Diphtheria, Tetanus, and Pertussis)
* IPV (Polio)
* MMR (Mumps, Measles, and Rubella).

A child was now receiving vaccinations for eight different diseases.

1970's - The only change to the immunization schedule was that the smallpox vaccine was no longer recommended due to its eradication. The number of vaccines that a child would receive actually went down by one for a total of seven.
* DPT (Diphtheria, Tetanus, and Pertussis)
* IPV (Polio)
* MMR (Mumps, Measles, and Rubella).

1980's and 1990's - Two more vaccines were introduced to the growing list of diseases that a child must be inoculated against. Children were being protected against nine different diseases.

- DTP (Diphtheria, Tetanus, and Pertussis)
- Hib (Haemophilus Influenzae)
- Hepatitis B

2000's - Changes to the immunization schedule continue to this day. More vaccines have been added to protect our children even further against infectious disease.

- DTaP (Diphtheria, Tetanus, and Pertussis)
- Hepatitis B
- IPV (Polio)
- MMR (Mumps, Measles, and Rubella).
- Hib (Haemophilus Influenzae)
- Hep A (Hepatitis A)
- PCV (Pneumococcus)
- RV (Rotavirus)
- MCV (Meningococcal)
- PPSV (Pneumonia)
- Varicella (Chicken Pox)
- There are currently other vaccines you can receive on a volunteer basis that include influenza, HPV (Human Papillomavirus), and the shingles vaccine.

The immunization schedule is always changing today. Your child will receive the majority of their vaccines by the time they are eighteen months old, with several being administered in one visit to the pediatrician. While I am not saying not to immunize your child, I am saying that you should be informed, ask questions, and research for yourself. My children have received all the vaccines required for their age. I am right there with you. With all these vaccines our children should be the healthiest generation to ever have lived. This is not so, is it? In fact, in my opinion, it is quite the opposite. This generation of children is probably the unhealthiest in terms of non-life threatening and debilitating chronic diseases, illnesses, and conditions.

Resources:

- CDC - INFO Contact Center #1-800-232-4636
- www.cdc.gov/vaccines
- To report a health problem that followed vaccination call the Vaccine Adverse Event Reporting System (VAERS) 1-800-822-7967
- Public tracking/listing of adverse reactions to vaccines go to http://vaers.hhs.gov/data/data
- The National Vaccine Information Center - www.nvic.org
- www.vaxtruth.org
- www.generationrescue.org/ (Autism Support Organization)
- Healing and Preventing Autism by Jenny McCarthy and Dr. Jerry Kartzinel
- www.immunize.org
- www.youtube.com/watch?v=Xwfnd_WRkiU
- www.naturalnews.com (go to the search bar on the top right of the home page and plug in vaccines. It will give you scores of articles on this topic)
- www.nvic.org (National Vaccine Information Center)

References

1. The Huffington Post, "Asthma Rates Rising, But Cause Unclear", Accessed in 2011, http://www.huffingtonpost.com/2011/05/04/asthma-rates-rising-but-c_n_857468.html

2. "FDA: Some chicken may have small amount of arsenic", Accessed June 8, 2011, http://www.huffibgtonpost.com/2011/06/08/arsenic-chicken_n_873299.html

3. Press TV,: Pesticide exposure in womb affects IQ", Accessed in 2011, http://www.presstv.ir/detail/176231.html

4. The New York Times, "Is Sugar Toxic", Accessed in 2011, http://www.nytimes.com/2011/04/17/magazine/mag-17sugar-t.html/?pagewanted=all

5. The New York Times, "Hiding the Truth About Factory Farms (editorial)", Accessed in 2011, http:/www.nytimes.com/2011/04/27/opinion/27wed3.html

6. "More Tainted Foods Coming From China", Accessed in 2011, http://voices.yahoo.come/more-tainted-foods-coming-china-5806590.html?cat=5

7. Kids Matter, "Kids not as healthy as parents think", Accessed in 2011, http://kidsmatter1.blogspot.com/2011/04/kids-not-as-healthy-as-parents-think.html

8. USA Today, "Pediatricians seek better regulation of toxins", Accessed in 2011, http://usa-today30.usatoday.com/news//health/medical/health/medical/pediatrics/story/2011/04/pediatricians-seek-better-regulation-of-toxins/46474962/1

9. USA Today, "Fight chronic illness in kids with preventive care", Accessed in 2011, http://usatoday30.usatoday.com/news/opinion/letters/2011-04-19-chronic-illness-in-children.htm

10. TribLive.com, "Energy drinks hot, medical jitters hotter", Accessed in 2011, http://triblive.com/x/pittsburgtrib/business/s_727975.html

11. Huffington Post, "Knew World's Best-Selling Herbicide Causes Problems, New Report Finds", Accessed in 2011, http://www.huffingtonpost.com/2011/06/07/roundup-birth-defects-herbicide-regulators_n_872862.html.

12. "Latest Toxic Toy Recalls: Lead and Cadmium in Toys and Jewelry", Accessed in 2013, http://www.babyrolls.com/49-latest-toxic-recalls-lead-and-cadmium-in-toys-and-jewelry

13. Huffington Post, "Painkillers, Antibiotics, Growth Hormones Among The 20 Chemicals found in typical Glass of Milk", Accessed on July 8, 2011, http://www.huffingtonpost.com/2011/07/07/milk=painkillers-antibiotics-hormones_n_892257.html

14. Psych Central, "Mice Study Finds Air Pollution Linked to Depression, Memory Issues", Accessed in 2011, http://Psychcentral.com/news/2011/07/06/mice-study-finds-air-pollution-linked-to-depression-memory-issues/27492.html

15. Natural News, "Is your food as healthy as you think?", Accessed on April 27, 2014, http://naturalnews.com/044865_healthy_food_heavy_metal_contamination_nutrition.html

16. Huffington Post, "Sugar-Sweetened Drinks Linked With High Blood Pressure", Accessed on April 27, 2014, http:///www.huffingtonpost.com/2014/04/24/sugar-drinks-blood-pressure_n_5208118.html

17. Huffington Post, "Think Dirty App Reveals Just How Toxic Certain Beauty Products Are", Accessed on April 27, 2014, http://www.huffingtonpost.com/2014/04/27/think-dirty-app-toxic_n_5212811.html

18. CNN, "Measles cases at highest level in nearly 20 years, CDC reports", Accessed on April 27, 2014, http://www.cnn.com/2014/04/24/health/measels-record-number/index.html

19. Fox News, "High-fat diets linked to some types of breast cancer", accessed on April 27, 2014, http://www.foxnews.com/health/2014/04/23/high-fat-diets-linked-to-some-types-breast-cancer/

20. Fox News, "1 in 3 children taking psychiatric medication in US", Accessed on April 27, 2014, http://www.foxnew.com/health/2014/04/25/1-in-13-children-taking-psychiatric-medication-in-us/

21. Natural News, "glyphosate found at high levels in mothers' breast milk", Accessed on April 28, 2014, http://www.naturalnews.com/044901_glyphosate_breast_milk_GMOs.htm

22. Forum on Child and Family Statistics, America's Children in Brief: Key National Indicators of Well-Being, 2010, Federal Interagency Forum on Child and Family Statistics, Katherine K. Wallman, Chief Statistician, Office of Management and Budget, http://www.childstas.gov/americaschildren

23. American Academy of Allergy Asthma and immunology, "Asthma", accessed on April 27, 2014, http://www.aaaai.org/conditions-and-treatments/asthma.aspx

24. Medline Plus, "Asthma in Children", Accessed on November 11, 2010, http://www.nlm.nih.gov/medlineplus/asthmainchildren.html

25. American Academy of Allergy Asthma and Immunology, "asthma statistics", Accessed on November17, 2010, http://www.aaaai.org/media/statistics/asthma-statistics.asp

26. Children and Adults with Attention Deficit and Hyperactivity Disorder, "What is AD/HD", Accessed on November 15, 2010, http://chadd.org/AM/template.cfm?section=understanding

27. Center for Disease Control and Prevention, "Data & Statistics", Accessed on April 27, 2014, http://www.cdc.gov/ncbddd/adhd/data.html

28. The Huffington Post, "ADHD Is on the Rise: How to Use Nutrition to Treat Attention Deficit", Accessed November 16, 2010, http://www.huffingtonpost.com/leo-galland-md/adhd-is-on-the-rise-_b_783381.html

29. National Institute of Mental Health, "Attention Deficit Hyperactivity Disorder" Accessed on April 27, 2014, http://www.nimh.nih.gov/health/topics/attention-deficit-hyperactivity-disorder-adhd/index.shtml

30. Autism Speaks, "What is Autism", Accessed on October 12, 2011, http://www.autismspeaks.org/what-autism

31. Autism Speaks, "What is Autism", Accessed on November 17, 2010 http://www.autismspeaks.org/whatisit/index.php

32. Autism Speaks, "Prevalence", Accessed on April 27, 2014, http://wwwautismspeaks.org/what-autism/prevalence

33. American Diabetes Association, "Statistics about Diabetes", Accessed on April 27, 2014, http://www.diabetes.org/diabetes-basics/staistics/

34. Center for Disease Control and Prevention, "Childhood Obesity Facts", Accessed on April 27, 2014, http://www.cdc.gov/healthyyouth/obesity/facts.htm

35. "Childhood Obesity Statistics", accessed on January 4, 2011, http://www.buzzle.com/articles/childhood-obesity-statistics.html

36. Center for Disease Control and Prevention, "Childhood Overweight and Obesity", Accessed on November 17, 2010, http://www.cdc.gov/obesity/childhhod/index.html

37. American Academy of allergy asthma and immunology, "Food Allergy", Accessed on December 6, 2010, http://www.aaaai.org/media/statistics/allergy-statistics.asp

38. Kids With Food Allergy A World of Support, "Food Allergy Among U.S. Children: Trends in prevalence and Hospitalizations" Accessed on October 20, 2010, http://www.kidswithfoodallergies.org/resourcespre.php?id=129&title=food_allergy_prevalence

39. Allergy Haven, Inc., "Food Allergy Basics", Accessed on December 6, 2010, http://www.allergyhaven.com/allergy_basics.htm

40. American Cancer Society, "What is Breast Cancer?", Accessed on December 3, 2010, http://www.cancer.org/cancer/breastcancer/detailedguide/breast-cancer-key-statistics

41. BreastCancer.Org, "U.S. Breast Cancer Statistics", Accessed on April 27, 2014, http://www.breastcancer.org/symptoms/understand_bc/statistics

42. Centers for Disease Control and Prevention, Immunizations: The basics, Accessed April 28, 2012, http://www.cdc.gov/vaccines/vac-g en/imz-basics.htm

43. Centers for Disease Control and Prevention, History of Vaccine Safety, Accessed on May 24, 2011, http://www.cdc.gov/vaccinesafety/vaccine_monitoring/history.html

44. Centers for Disease control and Prevention, Ingredients of Vaccines – Fact Sheet, Accessed on April 24, 2012, http://www.cdc.gov/vaccines/vac-gen/additives.htm

45. Centers for Disease Control and Prevention, Possible Side-effects from Vaccines, Accessed on May 1, 2012, http://www.cdc.gov/vaccines/vac-gen/side-effects.htm

46. Natural News, Health Basics: The 11 most toxic vaccine ingredients and their side effects by S.D. Wells, Accessed on May 1, 2012, www.naturalnews.com/z035431_vaccine_ingredients_side_effects_MSG.html

47. U.S. Department of Health and Human Services, Health Resources and Services Administration, National Vaccine Injury Compensation Program, Accessed on May 3, 2012, http://www.hrsa.gov/vaccinecompensation/index.html

48. U.S. Department of Health and Human Services, Health Resources and Services Administration, National Vaccine Injury Compensation Program statistical Reports, Accessed May 24, 2011, http://www.hrsa.gov/vaccinecompensation/data.html

49. Centers for Control and Prevention, Food and Drug Administration and U.S. Department of Health and Human Services, VAERS Data (vaccine adverse event reporting system), Accessed May 3, 2012, http://vaers.hhs.gov/data/index

50. VAERS (Vaccine Adverse Event Reporting system), Accessed May 3, 2012, http://www.vaers.hhs.gov/data/index

51. CBS News-Los Angeles, Study: US Quietly Paid Families For Vaccine-Linked Autism Cases, Accessed on May24, 2011, http:/losangeles.cbslocal.com/2011/05/11/study-us-quietly-paid-families-for-vaccined-linked-Autism-Cases/

52. National Vaccine Information Center, Vaccine Laws, Accessed April 30, 2014, http://www.nvic.org/vaccine-laws.aspx

53. National Conference of State Legislatures, States with Religious and Philosophical Exemptions From School Immunization Requirements, Accessed on April 30, 2014, http://www.nvic.org/research/health/school-immunizations-exemption-state-laws.aspx

54. The Children's Hospital of Philadelphia, Vaccine Education Center, Accessed on January 4, 2011, http://www.chop.edu/service/vaccine-education-center/vaccine-schedule/history-of-vaccine-schedule.html

55. The Centers for Disease Control and Prevention, 2014 Recommended Immunizations for Children from Birth Through 6 years old, Accessed May 1, 2014, http://www.cdc.gov/vaccines

CHAPTER 7
Chemicals in Our Daily Environment

"For the first time in the history of the world, every human being is now subjected to contact with dangerous chemicals, from the moment of conception until death."

—RACHEL CARSON

How many chemicals our children are exposed to on a given day depends on many lifestyle and environmental factors. One thing is for sure, they are exposed to far too many man-made, synthetic chemicals and toxins. Our bodies store these toxins and that toxic buildup leads to deficiencies, illness, and disease. According to the Merriam-Webster dictionary, the term chemical refers to a substance obtained by a chemical process or that produces a chemical effect. The chemical industry is one of the largest manufacturing industries in the United States and directly employs approximately 800,000 people.

According to the article, "The Great Chemical Unknown: A Graphical View of Limited Lab Testing", in 2010 there were roughly 50,000 chemicals used in consumer products and industrial processes. The article contends that only 300 have been tested for safety and only five have been labeled to have restricted use due to potential health concerns. In 2014, The Natural Resources Defense Council (NRDC) stated on its' website there is approximately 80,000 chemicals available in the United States that have never been fully tested for their toxic effects on our health and environment.

In 1976, The Toxic Substances Control Act (TSCA) was passed into law. The NRDC also believes this law has made it nearly impossible for the Environmental Protection Agency to take action against dangerous chemicals. The law, which has been in existence for over thirty years, has allowed thousands and thousands of chemicals into the products we use on a daily basis with limited testing and consequences for the chemical companies involved. Basically, no one knows what these chemicals are doing to our bodies and environment in the short and long term. Some of the chemicals produced can be found in: the shampoos, soaps, cosmetics, conditioners, cleaning products, toothpastes, antibiotics, over-the-counter medications, and foods we use and consume on a daily basis.

Chemicals are now being used to make just about everything we need or use on a daily basis. There are chemicals in the clothes that come back from the cleaners, in the furniture we buy, and the paints we use. There are chemicals in our carpeting and flooring, insect management sprays, toys, pots and pans, automobile parts, bug sprays, sunscreens, glues and solvents, batteries, perfumes, light bulbs, lawn and garden products, lipsticks and makeup, Tupperware, water bottles, hand sanitizers, medication and antibiotics, bedding, hair-coloring, cleaning supplies, and air fresheners. There are also chemicals in the water we drink and the air we breathe. We are exposed to chemicals and toxins from the moment we get out of bed in the morning until we lay our heads on the pillow at night. Let's look at an example of what I am referring to as it relates to our daily chemical exposure.

Example: The number of chemicals used in the example below is based on products that I purchased to indicate my point. They are all national brands and serve as a reference. The brands you potentially have in your home today may differ in terms of the number of ingredients or actual ingredients. However, I am confident that my ingredients will look pretty similar to yours.

Each morning, by the time you sit down for breakfast, you have already been exposed to hundreds of chemicals. How can that be you ask? Let's take a closer look.

- As you roll out of bed and gently lift yourself from your flame retardant mattress, (chemicals) you head straight to the bathroom. If you are a child, you are wearing flame retardant (chemicals) pajamas.

- Once in the bathroom, you brush your teeth. The toothpaste you use will have roughly fifteen synthetic chemical or chemical compounds including artificial colors, sweeteners, corn derivatives, thickening agents, fluoride, and emulsifiers (foam builders).

- The mouthwash you use will probably contain alcohol, artificial sweeteners, artificial colors, preservatives, and chemicals.

- Men who shave are exposed to more chemicals. These chemicals are directly applied to the biggest organ in your body, the skin.

- I count no less than twenty chemicals in my shampoo and approximately twenty in my conditioner. The soap I purchased is made up of fragrances (more chemicals), dyes, and emulsifiers. Your choice of body wash and soap is also made up of man-made chemicals. The water coming out of your shower head at a minimum contains fluoride, chlorine, heavy metals, and microorganisms.

- Once out of the shower, you reach for the towel that was washed in chemicals and dried with a chemical fabric softener.

- The deodorant you use will contain approximately ten different chemicals or chemical compounds including aluminum. If you use an aerosol spray, you will inhale these chemicals directly into your lungs as well as through your skin.

- Body lotion contains petroleum, emulsifiers, preservatives, alcohol, and chemical compounds.
- Women applying makeup every morning can include these toxins to the long list of chemicals you have been exposed to before you have left your bathroom to start your day.
- Perfume or cologne brings closure to the chemical barrage you just experienced getting ready for your day.

I am using this extremely exaggerated example to purposely highlight an important point. (I am not in fear of my bathroom and all of the products in it. I realize that by using less chemically laden products, I am simply reducing the amount of chemicals my family is exposed to on a daily basis.) The chemical barrage on your body begins the moment you wake up and never stops. Most of us never think about the chemicals we use on a daily basis to make ourselves feel and look physically attractive. While this example may seem extreme, and it is, remember this: while the chemicals used in the above illustration are used in small daily amounts, it is the cumulative effect these chemicals have on your body over time that you need to be aware of. One trip to the bathroom to get ready for your day equates to exposure to hundreds of man-made chemicals. I welcome you to the second barrage of chemicals during your morning when you sit down at the kitchen table for breakfast.

Take a few minutes and walk around your house. Pick up some cleaning products and read the labels. You will probably discover the ingredients are not even on the label. What is making your home smell fresh or helping to remove dirt from your toilets, floors, shower, and bathtubs? Open a drawer in your bathroom. Can you identify the ingredients in your toothpaste, mouthwash, or shampoo? I can hardly pronounce most of the ingredients, let alone know what they actually are.

Let's take a look at three items most of us use on a daily or weekly basis and that we have in our homes today. These are exaggerated examples that continue to highlight my point about chemicals. (I do not live in fear of sprays, light bulbs, or canned food. I know what some of the concerns are surrounding these items and I can now make an *informed* decision about whether or not I want to purchase them.)

I. **Disinfectant sprays:** I used to love to use a common household disinfectant spray in the past. I most often used this aerosol spray when my kids were little and one or all of them were sick. I would spray it in the air, on door handles, railings, sofas, and even their beds. I sprayed it everywhere! It claims to get rid of viruses, bacteria, mold, and even mildew. Disinfectant sprays will get rid of the most common germs lurking around a house full of children. It will sanitize the house and hopefully free the parent(s) of having to deal with the spread of germs to other family members. I loved it for years and thought it was a necessity to have a small arsenal at my fingertips. I picked up a can recently and actually read the label. The first thing I noticed was a precautionary statement on the label stating it is hazardous to humans and animals. It lists what to do in the event it gets on your hands or in your eyes. It even gives the phone number for the poison control center and warns that it is flammable. The one thing I could not find on the can was the list of ingredients. I called the phone number on the can to get some more information (This particular disinfectant spray, which was an original scent, is no longer available). I was told they do not list ingredients on the can because of spacing and marketing issues. The company would rather identify for the consumer all of the ways in which the product will help fight germs. I was also told they are not mandated by law to list the ingredients and that all labeling has been approved by the Environmental Protection Agency (EPA) and the Federal Drug Administration (FDA). I was verbally given the ingredient list over the phone and a website to further educate myself on the ingredients. Below are the ingredients found in one can of disinfectant spray:

- Ethanol, butane, and propane are the gases found in the ingredient list. All are flammable and can cause irritation to eyes and skin. Butane is a gas used to produce a "high" for people that choose to "sniff" it. It can cause euphoria, drowsiness, narcosis, asphyxia, and cardiac arrhythmia.
- Ethanolamine is a toxic, flammable, corrosive, and colorless liquid.
- Fragrance is a word used to describe the chemicals that give each scent its unique smell. The amount of chemicals will differ according to which scent you choose to purchase. I don't know what or how many chemicals are used to make a specific fragrance.

- Tetrasodium (EDTA), Sodium Benzoate, Myristalkonium Saccharinate, MEA Borate, and MIPA Borate are all chemicals and chemical compounds found in this particular disinfectant that act as preservatives, corrosion inhibitors, and complexing agents (Quite frankly, I would have to go back to school to begin to understand what I have just written).
- Ammonium hydroxide is yet another ingredient. It is basically a diluted form of ammonia which is used in most conventional cleaning products. Ammonia gives off a gas that can be toxic and will result in burning of the eyes, nose, and throat.
- Water. Oh, I forgot the last ingredient is water. I was politely reminded that water is a chemical. Give me a break!

This is a product that helps us prevent the spread of germs in our homes. What is the price we are willing to pay for germ-free homes? We are inhaling these chemicals directly into our lungs each and every time we spray them. There are several chemicals used in this one can and I believe it is safe to say that probably none of them have been tested for safety. There is nothing I can see from the ingredient list that is beneficial to our overall health. We are just spraying gases and chemicals in the air to mask and get rid of germs. The Natural Resources Defense Council conducted a study on fourteen different types of common household air fresheners. The study found that twelve of the fourteen air fresheners tested contain phthalates. Phthalates are hormone disrupting chemicals that can be dangerous to pregnant women and young children. Exposure to this chemical can affect testosterone levels and lead to reproductive abnormalities including abnormal genitalia and reduced sperm production. According to The Global Campaign for Recognition of Multiple Chemical Sensitivity, other chemicals used in air fresheners such as limonene, naphthalene, camphor, and dichlorobenzene are known toxins. Some are considered carcinogens and one is on the hazardous waste list. All of these chemicals effect the body in a negative way and over time can contribute to disruptions in health.

2. **The light bulb**: Our government has implemented regulations that the standard incandescent light bulb that has been used for more than one hundred years be phased out and replaced by the fluorescent or LED light bulb. We are told that the main

purpose for the switch is that the LED and fluorescent bulbs lasts longer and uses less energy. In other words, this bulb is environmentally friendly. Countries around the world including: Brazil, Venezuela, The European Union, Australia, Russia, Canada, Switzerland, and Argentina have already, or are currently in the process of, phasing out the incandescent bulb. How does the phasing out of the incandescent bulb affect you or more specifically your child? Well, the fluorescent light bulb contains mercury. Mercury vapor is released into the air when the bulb breaks. Mercury is a heavy metal that is toxic to humans. The Environmental Protection Agency (EPA) has outlined a three-page summary of cleanup guidelines should you be faced with a broken fluorescent bulb. It should be noted this guideline represents the *minimum* actions required to clean up the broken bulb. You can go to the website for updates on more effective cleanup practices as they become available (http://www2.epa.gov/cfl/cleaning-broken-cfl). The EPA website clearly states three steps for specific cleanup. The stages are outlined below.

Fluorescent light bulbs contain a small amount of mercury sealed within the glass tubing. When a fluorescent bulb breaks some of this mercury is released as mercury vapor. The broken bulb can continue to release mercury vapor until it is cleaned up and removed from the residence. The EPA recommends that residents follow the cleanup and disposal steps described below to minimize exposure to mercury vapor.

1. Before Cleanup:
- Have people and pets leave the room.
- Air out the room for five to ten minutes by opening a window or door to the outdoor environment.
- Turn off the heating or air conditioning system.
- Collect materials needed to clean up broken bulb.

2. During Cleanup:
- Be thorough in collecting broken glass and visible powder.
- Place cleaned-up materials in a sealable container.

3. After Cleanup:
- Promptly place all bulb debris outdoors in a trash container or protected area until materials can be disposed of properly. Avoid leaving any bulb fragments or cleanup materials indoors.

- If practical, continue to air out the room where the bulb was broken and leave the heating or air conditioning system off for several hours. Do not throw the broken bulb in your trash can outside. Broken fluorescent bulbs are considered hazardous and must be disposed of properly. The EPA website states you must check with your local or state government about disposal requirements in your area. Some states and communities require fluorescent bulbs (broken or unbroken) to be taken to a specific local recycling center.

This is another example of the toxins and chemicals that are so prevalent in our daily lives. We will save money on light bulbs because they last longer and require less electricity, but "Warning," they are hazardous to your health. We can take the necessary precautions and dispose of the bulb properly. Realistically speaking though, how many of us adults are:

- Aware that these bulbs contain mercury?
- Aware of the dangers of mercury (however small the amount)?
- Aware of how to properly dispose of these bulbs and at what location we can safely discard them?
- Going to actually and honestly take the time to dispose of these products at a proper facility?

My best guess is these bulbs are going in our trash cans whether they are broken or not. They will be thrown in the landfills with the other trash without regard to the potential hazard they pose to the environment or the health of individuals in a specific community. My other concern is what happens when your child breaks a light bulb and takes it upon themselves to clean up the mess because they just do not know any better?

The old incandescent bulbs are being phased out. In the coming years you will no longer be able to purchase them for private use in your own home unless a company finds a way to create an incandescent bulb that meets the new federal guidelines. At present, none of the incandescent light bulbs comply with the new federal law that requires a 30 percent cut in energy use. The bulbs will be phased out over a period of two years beginning in 2012 and ending in 2014. I highly recommend you be proactive about preparing your children with an evacuation plan in case of breakage of the new fluorescent bulbs. Children should never, ever get near a fluorescent bulb that is broken. Why are we putting mercury into something that is easily broken, used by children, and toxic to humans? Isn't it possible to create a more efficient bulb that does not contain mercury? Is it too much to ask that companies making this product inform consumers about this hidden danger? What is the harm in a company explaining this issue to its customers? Most of us will buy the bulb containing mercury because we have no choice. We have the right to be informed so we can take the necessary steps and educate our children on the dangers.

3. **The Aluminum Can:** I am referring to the aluminum can that soups, fruits, vegetables, pastas, and other side dishes come in and are found in almost every aisle of every grocery store. Not only do these cans appear in almost every aisle of the typical grocery store, but now the advertisements on the cans are being directly marketed to our children with images of Spiderman, SpongeBob SquarePants, princesses, Dora the Explorer, and more. What chemicals in the can allow or help the food or soup to maintain its freshness over a long period of time? The inside lining of the can is a different texture or color than the outside of the can. Why? I called and spoke to a representative from two leading soup companies to try to find out what, if any, chemicals are used to make this lining. It is important to know what chemicals are being used because the food that goes into these cans come into direct, constant contact with whatever chemicals are being used.

It occurred to me that the most important message I received from these companies is not the information they gave me over the phone. It is the information they would not give or share with me. Both companies stated that BPA (Bisphenol A) is used in making the inside lining of the can. I was assured that this chemical has been used for more than forty years throughout the food industry. Both companies also assured me their products were safe and that they were following the guidelines as outlined by the FDA. In trying to ascertain what other chemicals are being used to make the can I began to sense a "red flag" coming from both representatives. Either they did not have the information or they did not want to share the information with me. One company stated that due to proprietary issues they could not disclose such information. The other company passed along my contact information for another person to contact me. I have yet to receive a follow-up phone call. I am not sure how many years I have to wait for them to call me back? The only conclusion I can come up with is that these cans are lined with other chemicals, besides BPA, that may have harmful effects on your child's overall health.

I did a little more digging about chemicals used to make the can and found out some more interesting facts about the one ingredient that we now know is in the make-up of the aluminum can. BPA is a chemical used in manufacturing and is most recognized as a chemical used to make plastic water bottles. There has been a rise in awareness in the last few years on the part of consumers to purchase water bottles that are BPA free. BPA is a synthetic chemical that works to disrupt the important effects of estrogen in the brain. BPA's main purpose in aluminum food cans is to prevent the food product from reacting to the metal. BPA has already been shown to increase breast cancer cell growth. It has also been linked to a variety of health problems including: hormone disruption, prostate cancer, diabetes, obesity, and aggressive behavior in children. Scientific studies have connected BPA to cancer in animals as well as the development of fetal problems. It is my understanding that organic foods found in aluminum cans also contain BPA. I do know some companies are aware of the concern and are currently developing strategies to combat this problem.

I do not live in daily fear of beauty supplies, light bulbs, or aluminum cans. However, I think these three examples highlight the importance of the need for a better understanding of the daily environment our children are now exposed to in this country. The bigger question to me is what is the cumulative effect of these chemicals on a child's developing brain and body in the short and long-term? How are our children going to be affected throughout their lifetimes by a culture that promotes the use of chemicals in every facet of daily life? My common sense tells me they will be affected in a negative manner that does not serve their highest physical potential.

Before I switch gears and begin talking specifically about our food supply, below is a list of companies that sell beauty products with decreased amount of chemicals added to their products. The chemicals reduced or eliminated in these products may include: parabens, phthalates, petrochemicals, sulfates, silicone, synthetic fragrances, and dyes for color. Most of these products can be purchased at Target, Whole Foods, your local grocery store, and local health food stores. Most companies will carry a complete line of products to best meet your daily needs including: shampoo, conditioner, toothpaste, mouthwash, soap, eye cream, lip balm and glosses, sunscreen, facial towelettes, scrubs, lotions, foot cream, exfoliants, acne products, and body wash. The list of companies that are reducing the chemicals in their products is growing.

- Tom's
- Burt's Bees
- Alba Botanica
- Avalon Organics
- Jason
- Yes
- J, R, Watkins
- Dr. Bronner's
- Weleda
- GUD
- Eclos

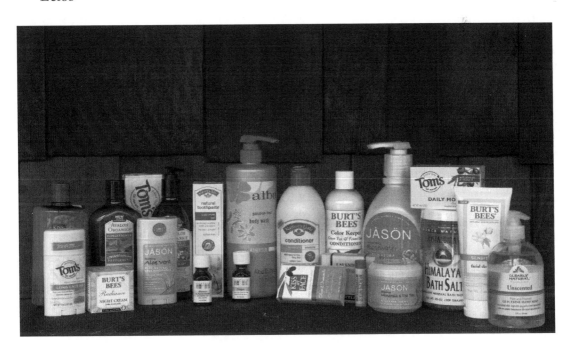

Remember that most cleaning supplies do not identify the ingredients on the bottle, so you really have no idea what you are using. Your skin is the biggest organ in your body. The chemicals found in most cleaning supplies are inhaled through your nose and mouth and ingested through your skin.

There are some organic or more natural products on the market today that do a good job of cleaning. They are much safer to use and contain far fewer chemicals than conventional options. These more natural cleaning products kill bacteria as well. The more natural, less toxic cleaning supplies listed below can be found at your local grocery store, Target, Wholefoods, and local health food stores. I was pleasantly surprised that Target carries a large selection of these supplies as well. These new products are comparable in price to most conventional cleaning supplies. You can also refer to the websites provided below to receive online coupons.

A good all-purpose cleaner eliminates the need for a large supply of products in your home and under your sink. I have eliminated countless bottles and sprays by using just a few products. The main idea is to find just a few chemically reduced products to replace your conventional cleaning supply needs. In the long run, you can save money by purchasing fewer supplies.

The main reason to change your cleaning supplies is to reduce or eliminate toxins including: chlorine, phosphorous, alcohol, formaldehyde, dioxane, animal products, perfumes, bleach, dyes, petrochemicals, and ammonia. Your new cleaning supplies will probably be non-flammable, non-toxic, non-abrasive, and possibly pH neutral. You will find that most of the ingredients will be derived from plants, essential oils, and are hypoallergenic.

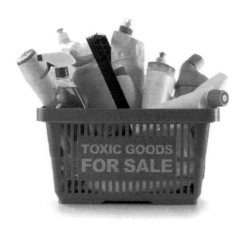

You will also find that companies are now making products that are more natural or organic in an attempt to tap into the organic marketplace. In 2010, U.S. consumers purchased $8.2 billion in natural and organic personal care products, representing a 6 percent increase in sales over the previous year. A company now sells both a highly processed and a less chemically laden version of the same item. For example, the all-natural toothpaste brand Toms is owned by Colgate-Palmolive. It is the same company with two very different toothpaste choices. Burt's Bees is now owned by the Clorox Company. The more natural Green Works cleaning supply product line is made by the Clorox Company. The Clorox Company dominates the shelf space for cleaning supplies and gives the consumer two separate and distinct choices. One choice is the conventional, chemically saturated cleaning supply. The second choice is a more natural, chemically reduced cleaning product. Why is the Clorox Company producing and marketing two different versions of the same product? Why did the Clorox Company purchase a more natural beauty care line in Burt's Bees? They are tapping into consumer demand. The Clorox Company understands the potential profit for their company if they develop and market products that are safer for everyone. Individuals are becoming more aware of the dangers of chemicals in their environment and are beginning to purchase products that reflect this mindset. Large corporations have no choice but to react to consumer spending trends.

I have also been able to find cleaning products that are less chemically saturated for laundry detergent, fabric softeners, bleach, dishwasher detergent, dish soap, toilet bowl cleaners, kitchen cleaners, window sprays, air fresheners, bathroom cleaners, toilet cleaners, all-purpose cleaners, surface wipes, and hand soap.

The brands that you can look for if you choose to eliminate some of the chemicals in your cleaning supplies include:

- Green Works (www.greenworkscleaners.com)
- Seventh Generation (www.seventhgeneration.com)
- ECOS and Earth Friendly Products (www.ecos.com)
- Green Shield Organics (www.greenshieldorganics.com)
- Citra-Solv, LLC (www.citra-solv.com)

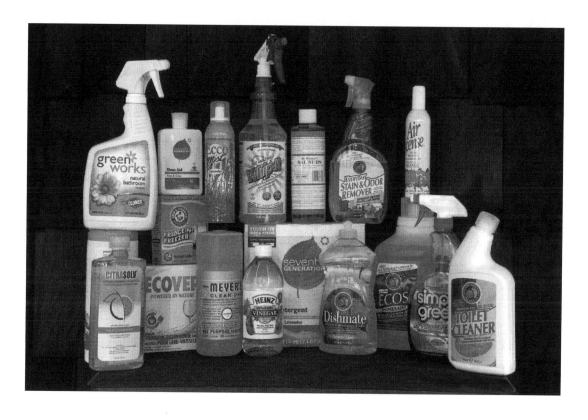

Take a minute to consider these questions:

1. How much antibiotic, steroid, pesticide, and hormone residue is in the chicken or beef you serve your family?

2. How much mercury is in the fish you serve?

3. Is the tap water you are serving your family and friends free of chemicals and toxins (fluoride, chlorine, heavy metals, etc.)?

4. Are the vegetables you are serving your children free of pesticides and chemical fertilizers?

5. Should you buy regular or organic foods? What is the difference and is it really beneficial?

6. Is the meat I am feeding my family corn-fed or grass-fed and what is the difference?

7. What about the milk? How many hormones and antibiotics were given to the cow for its milk now sits on my dinner table?

8. Why do some of the side dishes I serve my children have so many ingredients and what are they?

9. Do we really need that many preservatives in our food supply when thirty years ago we did not?

10. Why does most of what we eat have some type of corn derivative it in and why is that so important?

11. Did the chicken I am now serving ever see the light of day or was it cooped up in the hen house or cage with no windows and sunlight during its short life?

12. Why can food sit on the grocery market shelves for years?

13. What keeps the food in aluminum cans from spoiling?

14. Should I use the microwave oven even though it emits electromagnetic energy and radiation?

15. Should I use this plastic bottle if it is made from BPH or BPA?

16. Is sugar really that bad?

17. Why is soda unhealthy and what is phosphoric acid?

These questions never consciously entered my mind until a few years ago. I, like most parents, tried to watch what my kids ate and have always tried to encourage healthy eating habits. I wish I had been informed about true healthy eating years ago. It might have saved my son from years of needless heartache or at the very least minimized his physical symptoms. However, there is nothing I can do to change the past. I did the best I could at that time and am now more open to, educated about, and aware of our food, beauty, and cleaning product choices.

One of the biggest hidden dangers that exists for our children today is not the chemicals found in the garage, bathrooms, or under the sinks of most homes today (although this is important). The hidden danger that affects all of our children significantly and on a daily basis is the state of our current national food supply. The food that is purchased today that our children put directly into their growing bodies is filled with chemicals, pesticides, chemical fertilizers, fatty oils, preservatives, artificial ingredients, artificial colors, sugar, and artificial sweeteners. Some of this same food is now being genetically modified, if it is truly food at all.

It would be ridiculous for me to think I have the ability to rid my children's daily lives of all the chemicals found in their environment today. That is not my goal nor am I striving to achieve that outcome. However, I am doing my best to limit their daily exposure and trying to educate them and myself about some of the dangers. Decreasing the amount of chemicals found in cleaning products and beauty products is far easier to achieve than reducing the amount of chemicals currently found in food. Our family struggles with healthy food choices all the time. Our choices are not always ideal. We do the best we can individually and as a family. There are many times when I am not always sure if my children hear what I saying about the dangers, ignore what I am saying, or just don't care. I am OK, most of the time, with their responses for several reasons. I started to implement these changes at an age when they had already come to accept the "normal" dietary and societal habits we currently live in. I do believe I am passing on the groundwork that will empower them to make informed decisions. Ultimately though, the food choices they make now as teenagers and in the future are their own.

Aside from the chemicals found in food, it is important for all of us to understand that by genetically altering our food (GMO or Genetically Modified Organism) our children are more at risk of developing chronic illnesses now and in the future. It is my view that we are already seeing these negative consequences regarding the health of our children. We all know that cleaning supplies, gases, solvents, etc. are made up of chemical agents. Have you ever wondered what goes into the food that our kids eat every single day?

I had no idea the extent of this problem in my own home until one day I decided it was time to make some dramatic changes. I started by simply assessing the foods in the pantry closet, snack drawer, refrigerator, and freezer.

It became very clear to me that our entire family would have to participate in the transformation. Why not? We could benefit as well and support Frankie at the same time. I was beginning to understand that my household was getting ready for a major life change and shake-up. I had no idea how any of us were going to respond. I felt it was important enough to try. I made the decision to transform my kitchen and educate myself in the process. I have slowly changed my views on food. This transformation is no longer just about Frankie. It now concerns my entire family.

The remaining chapters in this section will take a closer look at some of the major problems in our food supply today. I believe you will be quite shocked to know what agricultural businesses are harvesting and what companies are putting into their products that are specifically marketed, advertised, and labeled with you and your child in mind. This is being done at your financial and physical expense.

References

1. Merriam-Webster, Definition of chemical, Accessed on May 1, 2014, http://www.merriam.com/dictionary/chemical

2. ICIS (market intelligence for the global chemical, energy and fertilizer industries), "Chemical industry employment levels continue to decline in the US and Europe", Accessed on May 1, 2014, http:k//www.icis.com/resources/news/2008/03/03/9104613/chemical-industry-employment-levels-continue-to-decline-in-the-us-and-europe

3. Scientific American, "The Great Chemical Unknown: A Graphical View of Limited Lab Testing", Accessed on May 1, 2014, http://www.scientificamerican.com/article/the-great-chemical-unknown/

4. National Resources Defend Council (NRDC), Take Out Toxics, Accessed on May 1, 2014, http://www.nrdc.org/health/toxics.asp

5. Lysol, Ingredient List, accessed on October 11, 2011, http://www.rbnainfo.com/productpro/productsearch.do?brandId=19&productLinedId=36

6. National Resources Defense Council (NRDC), "New Study: Common Air Fresheners Contain Chemicals That May Affect Human Reproductive Development", Accessed on November 17, 2011, http://www.nrdc.org/media/2007/070919.asp

7. The Global Campaign for Recognition of Multiple Chemical Sensitivity, "Let's Clear the Air about Air Fresheners and Plug-Ins", Accessed on November 17, 2011, www.mcs-america.org/airfresh.pdf

8. Consumer Reports, "Are incandescent bulbs being canned?", Accessed on May 18, 2011, http://www.consumerreports.org/cro/news/2010/08/q-a-are-incadescent-bulbs-being-canned/index.htm

9. United States Environmental Protection Agency (EPA), "What to Do if a Compact Fluorescent Light (CFL) Bulb or Fluorescent Tube Light Bulb Breaks in Your Home", Accessed on January 25, 2011, www.epa.gov/cfl/cflcleanup.pdf

10. Huffington Post, "BPA and Narrowed Arteries: New Study Links Plastics Chemical With Coronary Artery Stenosis", Accessed on August 16, 2012, http://www.huffington post. com/2012/08/15/bpa-narrowed-arteries-coronary-artery-stenosis_n_1783354.html

11. Organic Consumers Association, "Common Chemical Used in Food & Drink Packaging Causes Brain Damage in Children", Accessed on September 29, 2011, http://www.organic-consumers.org/foodsafety/bisphenolA120805.cfm

12. Rodale, "Canned Food Carries a Hidden Health Risk", Accessed on May 1, 2014, http://www.rodalenews.com/plastic-chemicals-and-canned-products

13. Huffington Post, "Burt's Bees, Tom's of Maine Owned by Fortune 500 Companies", Accessed on May 1, 2014, http://www.huffingtonpost.com/2012/04/20/burts-bees-toms-of-maine-green-products_n_1438019.htmlg

14. Organic Consumers Association, "Burt's Bees, Tom's of Maine, Naked Juice: Your Favorite Brands? Take Another Look", Accessed on May 1, 2014, http://www.organicconsumers.org/aticles/article_17306.cfm

CHAPTER 8
Problems with
the Food Supply

"If people let government decide what foods they eat and what medicines they take, their bodies will soon be in as sorry a state as are the souls of those who live under tyranny."

—THOMAS JEFFERSON

How bad can the food we are eating really be for us and our children? Let's take a look at some of the staple foods and how they are processed. There are several potential problems that can arise regarding chemicals and toxins hidden in the foods our children eat daily including some that are considered "healthy" for a growing body.

Before I talk about some of the dangers of the food supply today, I think it is important to highlight some of the recommendations made by the government in regard to our eating habits.

The food plate or pyramid highlights the governmental reommendations for daily nutritional intake for individuals. They both serve as a well-intentioned guide for a balanced daily diet.

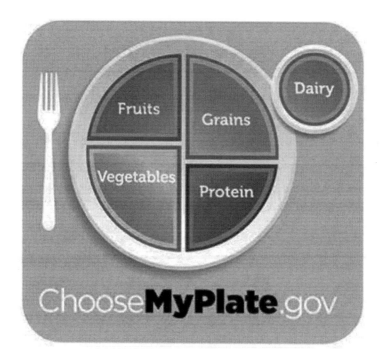

This food plate or pyramid clearly provides an example or standard of the types of foods that should be consumed on an on-going basis. While I think the government wants to educate the public about the many ways to enhance health through proper diet and nutrition, I am also suggesting that the typical and conventional foods being recommended have hidden dangers. On top of that, the proportion size for the different types of foods being recommended is out of balance and leans more toward acidic foods than alkalizing foods. We have the right to know what those hidden dangers are and become empowered to make necessary changes if we want. How bad can the food we are eating really be for us and our children? Let's take a look at some of the staple foods and how they are processed. There are several potential problems that can arise regarding chemicals and toxins hidden in the foods our children eat daily and that are considered "healthy" for a growing body.

Dairy/Beef

Understanding the change in, evolution of, and growing concerns about the ways in which milk and meat are produced in this country directly affects your family. Being empowered with the facts (on all sides) will allow you to make an informed decision.

The dairy and meat industries in this country are businesses that seek quick production and in large quantities. They have to because both industries are feeding millions of people each and every day. The production of milk and the raising of cattle is not the idyllic image of a farmer tending to a herd of cows grazing in the green pastures. Those days are long gone. How corporations produce these products in the U.S. has changed dramatically through the years. Today, small farms and farmers are being pushed out of the marketplace by the expansion of gigantic agricultural companies. It is getting harder and harder for the small farm to compete and stay alive today. Milk and meat are now being produced in mass quantities due to their daily demand from us.

Women have been providing their infants with breast milk to feed and provide necessary nutrients since the beginning of time. Today, women eventually wean their infants off of breast milk and introduce them to formula, store bought milk, baby food, and then regular food. This has been a natural process, but yet somewhere in this historical timeline, we have allowed children to continue milk consumption for the rest of their lives because it was thought to be good for them. I want to know who is giving us this information. Who spends millions of dollars yearly marketing milk? Well, my guess would be the companies that sell milk and the dairy farmers who produce the milk, who are subsequently subsidized by the U.S. government.

A subsidy is when government money (our money) is given to an organization or industry to help in its' overall function. From 1995-2012, the U.S. government subsidized the dairy industry $5.3 billion dollars. Taxpayers spend hundreds of millions of dollars a year subsidizing the dairy farmers due to government regulation and oversight. Of the $5.3 billion dollars we have personally contributed to this subsidy over a seventeen year period, how much of that money was spent researching, testing, and evaluating the chemicals that farmers are adding to their commodities that end up on our tables?

Not only is red meat difficult to digest, high in saturated fats, and can contribute to cardiovascular diseases, diabetes, high cholesterol levels, and cancer, but there are also other health concerns that you should be aware as it relates to the health of cows.

The large majority of cows are now raised on factory farms or feedlots with no beautiful pastures in which to roam. At a very young age cows are placed in confined spaces or feedlots and given antibiotics to ward off the diseases that typically increase given the type of environment they are now living in. The cows are also given hormones to speed up their production of milk. A cow's natural behavior is to graze in the pastures eating the grass that the land naturally provides. Grass has always been their main source of food. Most cows today no longer eat grass as their natural source of nutrition. It has been replaced by a grain-based corn diet.

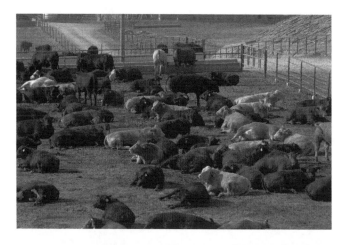

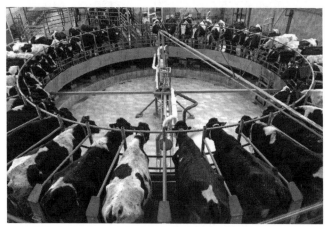

(Examples of different or average feedlots that can be found all across the country)

John Robbins is a national speaker and author on healthy living. He turned down the opportunity to run his father's business, Baskin's Robbins, in search of his own life's destiny. According to John Robbins, seventy-five years ago steers lived to be four or five years old at slaughter. Today, they are fourteen to sixteen months old. You can't take a beef calf from eighty pounds at birth to 1,200 pounds in a little more than a year on grass. It takes enormous quantities of corn, protein supplements, antibiotics, and other drugs including growth hormones. Mr. Robbins also maintains that the heightened prevalence of E. coli bacteria is a direct result of the commercial meat industry's practice of factory farming and the introduction of corn into the cow's diet. He is not the only one to assert this claim. We have created an unhealthy cow by changing their diet, injecting them with steroids, antibiotics, and growth hormones, and confining them to cramped and dirty living conditions.

There is no positive health or nutritional benefit for the cow or us to switch a cow's diet from grass to grain (corn) that I am aware of today. Grain-fed cows suffer from more disease and sickness because grains are not processed as easily or as naturally as grass in their digestive system. It is cheaper in the long run for companies to feed cattle ready-to-eat grains than it is to maintain land for the cattle to roam. It is more cost productive for producers to keep animals confined in a small space, accelerate the age at which you can slaughter them for meat or produce increased quantities of milk.

One of the main goals of the slaughterhouses and dairy producers is to get the cow up to slaughter or dairy weight as fast as possible. The idea is to get the cow to produce as much milk as efficiently and effectively as possible. These industries do not differ in regard to other societal institutions and norms. Most companies and industries produce a product for a profit. The bottom line is what keeps companies motivated. In 1950, the average dairy cow produced 5,300 pounds of milk a year. In 2011, a typical cow produced more than 18,000 pounds of milk. An average dairy cow in 2014 produced approximately 21,000 gallons of milk.

One of the ways that dairy farmers achieve this outcome is by giving the cows a growth hormone called Recombinant Bovine Growth Hormone (rBGH) or Recombinant Bovine Somatotropin (rBST). This is a genetically engineered hormone made in a laboratory that is given to the cow to increase milk production. We are replacing naturally occurring hormones in cows and humans with synthetic, man-made hormones. This cannot be good for us or the cow?

Just to summarize, cows are now confined to unsanitary living conditions, we have switched what they are eating, are giving them synthetic hormones to accelerate natural maturation rates, and are now providing them with increased amounts of antibiotics to ward off disease and sickness. Dairy cows today are more prone to develop mastitis, an infection of the udder that requires an antibiotic, because of the huge amounts of milk they are forced to produce. Mastitis will leave the cow's udder swollen and bleeding with pus that sometimes is excreted into the milk. Antibiotics given to cows or humans work the same way. The antibiotic kills both the good and bad bacteria. When given too many antibiotics, the cows will develop a resistance to the antibiotic. The bacteria will continue to thrive in the cow and more and more antibiotics are needed. It is a cyclical nightmare for the cow.

FDA approval for rBST or rBGH (recombinant bovine growth hormone) came in 1993 despite strong opposition from some scientists, farmers, and consumers. It was also the first major biotechnology food product approved by the FDA. A USDA study in 2007 found that 1 in 5 (17%) cows were being injected with rBGH, while another study has that number at 22%.

According to detractors, rBGH was never properly tested. The FDA relied solely on a study done by Monsanto, the same company who engineered and patented rBGH. The study conducted tested the safety of rBGH for human consumption. The study took all of ninety days to complete and used thirty rats to assess the results that would inevitably affect millions and millions of people. The study was never published and the FDA stated the results showed no significant problems. A review by a Canadian health agency on rBGH found that the ninety day study showed a significant number of issues which should have triggered a full review by the FDA.

The hormone rBGH is banned in countries including Japan, Canada, Australia, and the entire European Union. The United States cannot export its beef to some of these countries. Their laws have mandated that no beef be injected with rBGH due to health concerns. It is hard to know what the long-term effects of rBGH are on humans. If you take a look at some of the problems that the cows are enduring, then one can only make the conclusion that there is a potential risk to us and our children.

Some of the problems associated with rBGH in regard to the cow's health are an increase in mastitis, an increase in hoof diseases, open sores, and bovine death stemming from internal bleeding. A 1991 report by Rural Vermont highlights that cows that are forced to produce unnaturally high quantities of milk will often become malnourished. The cow loses more nutrients through their milk than they are ingesting in their feed. This makes them more susceptible to disease. Milk from rBGH-treated cows contains higher levels of IGF-1 (Insulin Growth Factor-1). Humans also naturally have IGF-1 and increased levels in humans have been linked to colon and breast cancer. The American Cancer Society has taken a look at the health concerns regarding rBGH and increased IGF-1 levels in humans. While their findings are inconclusive in regard to human safety, it is evidenced that cows are not doing so well.

Robyn O' Brien, in her book, *The Unhealthy Truth*, has uncovered some startling facts about the "revolving door" as she puts it. I will give you one example of her research and highly suggest that you get a copy of her book. She is a mother whose child experienced a life threatening food allergy. She has taken the initiative to speak out about the problems associated with the food industry today. She does an extraordinary job of highlighting and bringing to the forefront all that is wrong and a cause for concern. Through her extensive research, she discovered that The FDA's deputy commissioner at the time of approval for rBGH was a man named Michael Taylor. Before joining the FDA, he worked at a law firm that handled all of Monsanto's legal work. Mr. Taylor had represented Monsanto while the company was seeking FDA approval of rBGH. Mr. Taylor left the FDA after overseeing the regulatory approval of rBGH and was hired back to be vice president of public policy for Monsanto. Robyn O'Brien gives example after example of people who worked both for Monsanto and the U.S. government. I hate to highlight the fact that no one is looking out for your family but I will. Well, at least not the people you probably think should be.

The government approved a synthetic hormone under scrupulous conditions to a company doing everything in its power to close or eliminate all small farms in this country. Monsanto uses a synthetic hormone that we end up ingesting and which some say increases cancer risks and produces a host of questionable health concerns. This Company worked tirelessly to promote its new growth hormone and used political clout, money, and lobbying efforts to squash or hinder efforts by others to bring legitimate concerns about its safety to the forefront.

I have learned I can greatly reduce or eliminate my family's dairy intake while finding alternative foods for calcium absorption. That is after all the main reason we think our children need milk right? I have always been told that milk provides the nutrients (calcium) to make our bodies and bones strong. It is a correct statement that our bodies need calcium. Calcium is a mineral and a building block for our bones. Is it possible to find other food sources that provide calcium and do not pose a health risk to us or our children?

The evolution of milk production and its hidden dangers go deeper than what I have outlined above. The milk found in most grocery stores is pasteurized and homogenized as well.

Pasteurization is a process of heating milk to a certain temperature for a certain amount of time. This process kills the microorganisms that may cause us potential harm. Milk is heated to a temperature of approximately 161 degrees for 15 seconds during this process. Ultra-pasteurization requires heating the milk to a temperature of approximately 280 degrees for a second or two. This is also done to promote a longer shelf life.

The process of homogenization is used to separate the fat from the liquid which results in a smooth texture. In the process of heating the milk, vital nutrients made up of enzymes, vitamins, minerals, and good bacteria are destroyed. The milk has to then be fortified with synthetic vitamins due to the loss of naturally occurring ones. It is important to understand that organic milk is also pasteurized. Organic milk production by law has to also follow the same guidelines established by the federal government for the regulation of all milk production in this country. Organic milk is however free from artificial hormones (including rBGH), antibiotics, and other chemicals. The cows are supposed to only consume certified, organic feed. In 2010, the USDA closed a loophole in their organic regulations.

All organic dairy cattle must now spend much of the year grazing in open pastures as opposed to feedlots. Our federal government is conducting swat-style raids on small farms all across this country in an effort to eliminate their perceived enemy,

American citizens who are choosing to drink unpasteurized and unprocessed milk. We are willing to punish people for drinking raw milk, but have no qualms about drinking milk that has been significantly altered in many ways. For a timeline of federal raids on small farms you can go to http://naturalnews.com/033280_FDA_raids_timeline.html for more information.

The average person in the U.S. consumes 3 hamburgers a week and more meat in general than any other people in the world. The industrialization of our meat industry is also a cause for concern and a better understanding might be helpful for the public at large. The industrialization of the meat supply (chicken, beef, and pork) has led to innovation, new technologies, and improved efficiencies in terms of meeting production demands. What we are failing to see is that the product is contaminated and we know that can lead to a toxic (acidic) buildup in our bodies.

Here are some of the positive and negative aspects of factory farmed cows and grass-fed cows.

Factory Farmed Cows/Beef	**Grass-Fed Cows/Beef**
Digestive issues as a result of a corn fed diet	No digestive problems as a result of diet
Cost to customer is cheaper	Cost to customer is more expensive
Higher in saturated fats and lower in omega-3 fats	Lower in saturated fats and higher in omega 3
Lower in nutrients	Higher in Vitamin E and linoleum content
Dependence on petroleum	Less dependence on petroleum
Cows live in unsanitary and confined conditions	Less unsanitary conditions
Cows injected with antibiotics and steroids	Not injected with antibiotics and steroids
Produce more methane gas and manure	Requires more land to roam

There are significant environmental problems or concerns associated with factory farmed cows and grass-fed cows. However, grass-fed cows are the healthier option to prepare and eat for you and your family.

I suggest watching the movie Food, Inc. if you want to better understand what is happening in regard to the production of meat in this country. It is a good starting point and lays out the problems and health issues that the cows are now faced with. It also connects the meat industry's problems to our own health.

Keep in mind that we have not even discussed what preservatives are added to the meat for packaging and selling purposes. There are several preservatives used in the food industry today to ensure that your beef, poultry, and pork stay "fresh" for a longer length of time. These preservatives will decrease bacteria, fungi, and parasites.

Beef, poultry, and pork all have a short shelf life. This means that they are a perishable item and if not eaten in a certain amount of days they will begin to spoil and decay. Whether you are purchasing beef, pork, chicken, deli meats, or processed meats there are a few preservatives that I keep reading about. There are three previously banned preservatives that have now been approved by a division of the USDA for use. They are sodium benzoate, sodium propionate, and benzoic acid. You can also find nitrites and nitrates, sulphites, meat glue, viral sprays, and carbon monoxide treatments used in the preservation of meat. Fresh chicken also has the potential to contain the following preservatives: sodium and potassium lactate, bromelain, MSG, and ficin.

Another practice on the rise which potentially has unintended consequences to our health is the process of irradiation. The process of irradiation is basically another tool the meat industry uses to decrease the amount of bacteria found on meat. We can also routinely kill bacteria found in our meats by heating, freezing, or treating this product with a chemical. Irradiation does not eliminate the bacteria problem completely. We are told it helps to control unwanted organisms in our meat supply.

The United States has been experimenting with food irradiation for more than thirty years and more specifically, since after World War II. The process of irradiation exposes the meat to low levels of radiant energy and radiation. The USDA has determined that this practice is safe because it does not expose humans to increased radiation. We are told the radiant energy used is not strong enough and does not come into direct contact with the food. Other countries such as Canada, Sweden,

Denmark, and the United Kingdom also suggest this practice is safe. Food irradiation has also received endorsement from the World health Organization, The American Medical Association, and the International Atomic Energy Agency. We are also told this procedure does not change the nutritional value of the meat and poses no health consequences to humans. Irradiation treatment is currently used in the food industry as a preservative, to sterilize certain foods, to control food-borne illnesses, and to control sprouting, ripening, and insect damage. In addition to certain foods being irradiated, this process is also being used in The United States for performing security checks on hand luggage at the airports, making tires more durable, making non-stick cookware coatings, purifying wool, and destroying bacteria in cosmetics. Food irradiation is overseen by the USDA. Since 1986 all irradiated foods must carry this international symbol called a Radura.

The main motive for irradiating meat is a financial one. If foods are prevented from spoiling or their ripening is delayed these foods can sit longer on grocery store shelves. It also means they can be shipped to greater distances.

Consumer groups are concerned because irradiating a food product can give the consumer the perception that a perishable product is still fresh which potentially puts the consumer at risk. Another concern being debated is whether or not the nutritional value of the product is manipulated. Some groups also question the potential health risks to humans in the long term. I do not recall ever seeing this label on the packaging of the food I purchased in the past. I would surmise this issue is just something to be aware of as you shop for your family. My thought is if a food product has to be irradiated, maybe I don't want to buy it all! Below is a chart identifying potential food irradiation uses and their potential effects on specific foods:

Type of food	Effect of Irradiation
Meat, poultry	Destroys pathogenic organisms
Perishable foods	Delays spoilage, retards mold growth, and reduces number of microorganisms
Grain, fruit	Controls insects in vegetables and infestations in dehydrated fruit, spices, and seasonings, reduces rehydration time
Onions, carrots, potatoes, garlic, ginger	Inhibits sprouting
Bananas, mangos, papayas, guavas, other non-citrus fruits	Delays the ripening

Recommendations for you or your family:

- Try almond or coconut milk instead of dairy milk
- Purchase organic milk and cheese
- Reduce the overall amount of milk and cheese consumed
- Consider alternatives to processed cheese
- Purchase organic meats and grass-fed beef
- Reduce the amount of meat you eat on a weekly basis
- The only way to eliminate irradiated food products is to buy organic. According to the United States Department of Agriculture guidelines, any product that bears the certified organic seal cannot be treated with irradiation. This applies to every ingredient included in a specific product.

It is important to know how much calcium your body requires on a daily basis. Below is a chart that specifies the amount of calcium needed per day based on age.

Life Stage	Recommended Amount
Birth to 6 months	200 mg
Infants 7–12 months	260 mg
Children 1–3 years	700 mg
Children 4–8 years	1,000 mg
Children 9–13 years	1,300 mg
Teens 14–18 years	1,300 mg
Adults 19–50 years	1,000 mg
Adult men 51–70 years	1,000 mg
Adult women 51–70 years	1,200 mg
Adults 71 years and older	1,200 mg
Pregnant and breastfeeding teens	1,300 mg
Pregnant and breastfeeding adults	1,000 mg

Broccoli, kale, green beans, cabbage, sweet potato, celery, chick peas, carrots, spinach, onion, cauliflower, almonds and almond butter, sesame, chia and flax seeds, brazil nuts, kiwi, figs, dates, apricots, oranges, tangerine, raisins, sardines, salmon, kidney beans, French beans, olives, basil, thyme, sage, oregano, and dill all provide calcium. You can also buy organic products that are fortified with calcium. This list is not exhaustive as other fruits and vegetables contain smaller amounts of calcium. Grains provide only a small amount of needed calcium and are not included in the above list.

If you would like to reduce the amount of animal protein you are consuming, below are suggestions of foods high in protein.

Beans (kidney, white, lima, black, and mung), seeds (flax, chia, hemp, sesame, pumpkin, and sunflower), eggs, tuna (would avoid canned Tuna), salmon, halibut, haddock, pasta, asparagus, couscous, goji berries, squash, nuts (minus cashews and peanuts because they have higher levels of mold than other nuts), bananas, Brussels sprouts, carrots, cauliflower, strawberries, quinoa, brown rice, avocados, broccoli, artichokes, and oatmeal. Again, this list is not exhaustive. There are certainly other fruits, vegetables, legumes, and grains that contain smaller amounts of protein. There are also plant protein powders available that can be added to water or smoothies.

References

1. Disabled World, "Old and New Food Pyramid with Pictures", Accessed on May 3, 2014, http://www.disabled-world.com/artman/publish/food_pyramid.shtml

2. United States Department of Agriculture, My Plate Graphic Resources, Accessed on May 3, 2014, http://www.choosemyplate.gov/images/myplateimages/jpg/myplate_green.jpg

3. Environmental Working Group, Farm Subsidy Database, Accessed on May 3, 2014, http://farm.ewg.org/progdetail.php?fips=00000&progcode+dairy

4. John Robbins, "What About Grass-fed Beef", Accessed on August 2, 1011, http://www.johrobbins.info/blog/grass-fed-beef/

5. Grace Communications Foundation, Hormones, Accessed on January 24, 2011, http://www.sustainabletable.org/258/hormones

6. Dairy Moos, How much milk do cows give?, Accessed on May 5, 2014, http:/www.dairy-moos.com/how-much-milk-do-cows-give/

7. Grace Communications Foundation, rBGH, Accessed on August 4, 2011, http://www.sustainabletable.org/issues/rbgh/

8. Grace Communications Foundation, rBGH, Accessed on May 7, 2014, http://www.sustainabletable.org/797/rbgh

9. American Cancer Society, Recombinant Bovine Growth Hormone, Accessed on May 5, 2014, http:www.cancer.org/cancer/cancercauses/othercarcinogens/athome/recombinant-bovine-growth-hormone

10. About.com Guide, "Why are factory farmed animals given antibiotics and hormones such as rBGH?", Accessed on January 24, 2011, http://animalrights.about.com/od/animalsusedforfood/f/antibioticsrGBH.htm

11. SourceWatch.org, RBGH, Accessed on August 4, 2011, http://www.sourcewatch.org/index.php/rbgh

12. Robyn O'Brien, The Unhealthy Truth, [New York: Broadway Books, 2009]

13. Organic Valley, "Pasteurization Processes of Organic Valley Milk", Accessed on May 5,2014, http://www.organicvalley.coop/products/milk/pasteurization/Natural News, "The Facts About Pasteurization and Homogenization of Dairy Products", Accessed on May 5, 2014, http://www.naturalnews.com/022967_milk_pasteurization_dairy.html

14. About.com Guide, "Organic Milk vs. Regular Milk: Udderly Superior", Accessed on May 7, 2014, http://greenliving.about.com/od/greenshopping/a/organic-milk.htm

15. Natural News, "USDA canes to food industry pressures, approves three new toxic meat preservatives", Accessed on January 14, 2014, http://www.naturalnews.com/039792_USDA_meat_preservatives_chemicals.html

16. Steven Knapp, A summary of the PBS special called: "Modern Meat: A PBS Frontline documentary", Accessed on November 17, 2010

17. About.com Guide, "What are Feedlot Beef, Organic Beef and Grass-Fed Beef?", Accessed on January 14, 2014, http://animalrights.about.com/od/animalsusedforfood/a/GrassFedBeef.htm

18. Corn Fed Beef vs Grass Fed Beef, Accessed on September 22, 2010, http://www.deathfood.com/cornfedbeef.htmln

19. Idaho State University, "Ten Most Commonly Asked Questions About Food Irradiation", Accessed on January 15, 2014, http://www.physics.isu.edu/radinf/food.htm

20. UW Food Irradiation Education Group, What is Food Irradiation, Accessed on January 14, 2014, http://www.uw-food-irradiation.engr.wisc.edu/Facts.html

21. LoveToKnow Organic, Irradiated Foods, Accessed on May 22, 2011, http://www.organic.lovetoknow.com/food_irradiation

22. Mindfully.org, The Truth about Irradiated Meats, Accessed on January 14, 2014, http://www.mindfully.org/Food/2003/Irradiated-Meat-TruthAug03.htm,

23. National Institutes of Health, Calcium, Accessed on May 7, 2014, http://ods.od.nih.gov/factsheets/Calcium-QuickFacts/

CHAPTER 9
Corn, Corn, Corn, and So Much More

"When planning for a year, plant corn. When planning for a decade, plant trees. When planning for a life, train and educate people."

—CHINESE PROVERB

Corn: This is the hidden commodity found in almost all food and cosmetic items you have in your house today. The Unites States is the largest producer of corn in the world. In 2000, corn was grown on over 400,000 farms all across this country. From 1995-2012, the U.S. Government subsidized the corn industry $84.4 billion dollars. So much corn is now being produced there have been creative and scientific breakthroughs in the way it can be incorporated into the production of food and more specifically, processed foods. If you take a look at the ingredient list of almost all food items you buy for your children, chances are high that corn or one of its' many derivative will be on the list.

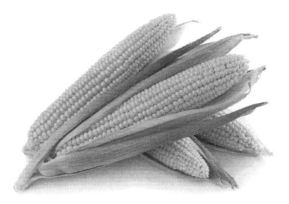

There has been much debate in the last few years about the effect this ingredient has on our overall health. I had no idea about the potential hidden risks associated with commercially farmed corn until a few years ago. I did not know corn could even be engineered into other ingredients or derivatives and why this might be harmful.

Corn can be used several different ways. It can be turned into ethanol, left alone as simple corn on-the-cob, used as feed for animals, or turned into several differently named ingredients that are used in most foods we consume today. While some will argue that corn has some health benefits including certain vitamin B, folate, fiber, and phosphorous, the amount of corn being consumed is a hidden danger. I will also suggest those healthy nutrients can be found in corn before it has been altered and loses those nutritional benefits. We will focus on two key areas related to corn: high fructose corn syrup (HFCS) and corn derivatives.

High fructose corn syrup (HFCS) is a derivative of corn and is substituted in most packaged foods today as an alternative to sugar. It is a replacement for sugar because it is plentiful and cheaper to produce. To put this into context, the average person today consumes approximately 140 pounds of HFCS and sugar. One hundred years ago the average person consumed approximately 4 pounds of sugar and ten thousand years ago an individual consumed 20 teaspoons of sugar a year. The consumption of

HFCS has increased 1000% between 1970 and 1990. HFCS is a product that is cheaply made, debatably unhealthy, and contributing not only to obesity, but too many conditions we see in adults and children today including: diabetes, liver disease, metabolic syndrome, neurotoxicity, heart disease, stroke, cancer, and inflammation. The increased use of HFCS in the United States mirrors the rapid increase in obesity. High fructose corn syrup is an industrialized ingredient and is extracted from corn stalks through a chemical enzymatic process. We know every type of sugar can be reduced or eliminated as much as possible from our diets. However, there is a distinct and important difference in the way our bodies digest HFCS as compared to cane or white sugar.

What is the difference between cane sugar (sucrose) and corn sugar (HFCS)?

Cane sugar and corn sugar is not the same thing, nor does the body digest them the same way. According to an article published by the American Journal of Clinical Nutrition, the digestion, absorption, and metabolism of fructose differ from those of glucose. The white "everyday" sugar we use most often today is refined cane sugar (sucrose). Both "everyday" white sugar and cane sugar are made up of two sugar molecules bound tightly together in equal amounts (50–50). These molecules are glucose and fructose. Your digestive tract breaks down the sugar (sucrose) into glucose and fructose which are absorbed into the body. HFCS is also made up of glucose and fructose but not in equal amounts (45–55) and in an unbound form. Fructose is sweeter than glucose, thus HFCS has a sweeter taste based on the ratio of glucose to fructose. Since there is no chemical bond between them, the body does not digest HFCS. It is rapidly absorbed into the blood stream once consumed. The fructose will head straight to the liver and the glucose triggers immediate spikes in insulin. These two results of HFCS lead to potential increases in metabolic disturbances that increase appetite, weight-gain, diabetes, heart disease, cancer, liver damage, dementia, hypertension, and elevated "bad" cholesterol levels. Another cause for concern in regard to HFCS is the prevalence of mercury. According to an article in USA TODAY, almost half of the tested samples of commercialized high fructose corn syrup contained mercury. Again, mercury is toxic to humans.

Anytime a product contains HFCS you can bet there are other chemicals including preservatives and food dyes. It is almost always found in food products that are nutritionally depleted. As people become more aware of the potential health problems associated with HFCS, the corn industry and possibly the U.S. government will begin ramping up their marketing campaigns to highlight the benefits of this product. The corn industry is calling into question anyone who claims this product is harmful. They also claim that HFCS and sugar are the same. They are not. Don't take my word for it. Research this topic on your own and come up with your own answers. The corn industry is also reaching out to the medical community asserting that this ingredient is safe. Why? The answer is simple. It comes down to money and making as much as possible. When you are looking at the ingredients of a product in the grocery store be aware of the following ingredients because they are derivatives of corn.

Tocopheryl	Mannitol	Sorbitol
Vanilla extract	Maltodextrin	Malt
Corn starch	Corn oil	Xanthan gum
Dextrose	Malt syrup	Corn flour
Corn meal	Dextrin	Mono- and- diglycerides
Malt extract	Corn syrup	Lactic acid
Sodium sitrate	Calcium citrate	Malitol
Vinegars	Cellulose	Potassium citrate
Citric acid	Citrate	Treacle

How many products actually contain HFCS or one of its' many derivatives? How widespread is this potential health problem? I recently conducted an experiment and headed off to my local grocery store. I went up and down each and every isle reading the ingredients of well-known conventional food brands and products that can be found at every grocery store across this country. Below are the lists I was able to compile. I subdivided the lists into two groups. I am sure I missed many products that contain HFCS or a corn derivative, but I am sure you can see the point that I am trying to convey. The first list is the foods that specifically state high fructose corn syrup as an ingredient and the second list contains names of different types of corn derivatives found in most packaged foods. Often a product will carry both HFCS and one or more of its derivatives.

PRODUCTS CONTAINING HIGH-FRUCTOSE CORN SYRUP:

- Jelly
- Yogurt
- Frozen juices
- Popsicles
- Frozen and packaged breakfast foods including waffles, pancakes, and breakfast sandwiches
- Ice cream
- Breads, bagels, frozen rolls, and garlic toast
- Chocolate syrup
- Most frozen prepared meals and entrees
- Pickles
- Packaged cakes, donuts, cinnamon rolls, and coffee cakes
- Toddler fruit bars
- Antacid and calcium supplements (liquid and tablets)
- Dog and cat food
- Children's cough medicine
- Children's fever reducing medications
- Night-time cold and flu medicine for adults
- Cough drops
- Marshmallows
- Most packaged cookies that are sold in either individual bags or one big package
- Animal crackers
- Bottled teas

- Cinnamon graham crackers
- Canned baked beans, kidney beans, black-eyed peas, diced tomatoes, plum tomatoes, and some vegetables and fruits
- Boxed potatoes with cheese sauce
- Condiments including: ketchup, barbeque sauce, pickle relish, Dijon mustard, and bottled marinades
- Crackers (white and wheat, peanut butter, and cheese-filled)
- Lollipops, hard candies, gummy bears and worms, chewy candy, packaged fruit-strips and fruit pieces, boxed cakes, frostings, and muffins
- Pop-tarts and breakfast bars
- Sugar cereals
- Sports drinks
- Soda
- Lemonade

PRODUCTS WITH DERIVATIVES OF CORN ON INGREDIENT LIST:

- Ice cream cones
- Peanut butter
- Liquid eggs
- Prepackaged rolls
- Margarine
- Frozen French fries
- Frozen vegetables with sauce
- Frozen desserts
- Fish sticks
- Hot dogs
- Bologna

- Packaged chicken nuggets
- Children's vitamin
- Deodorant
- Children's flavored toothpaste
- Regular toothpaste
- Supplemental liquid nutritional drinks
- Fiber pills
- Children's flavored fever-reducer
- Shampoos, soaps, and conditioners
- Cheese balls
- Gum
- Artificial sweeteners
- Pretzels and chips (baked and fried)
- Pancake mixes
- White and butterscotch cookie chips
- Packaged puddings
- Ginger ale and flavored seltzer waters
- Tortilla chips
- Boxed oatmeal
- Granola bars
- Bottled salsa
- Salad dressings
- Boxed, seasoned rice, and pasta side dishes
- Macaroni and cheese
- Soup in cans and boxes
- Olives
- Mayonnaise

A large and growing number of processed food products found in the aisles of your local grocery store are filled with high fructose corn syrup and other corn derivatives. Don't forget the meat we consume on a daily basis and the cosmetic and toiletry items we use also have derivatives of corn. Our bodies are now being overwhelmed with a product that is not digested naturally. This generation of children is the first ever in the history of the world to be inundated and barraged by corn, its' derivatives, and the many possible health consequences. Most of the foods listed above are loaded with not only HFCS or corn derivatives, but with preservatives, added salt, artificial colors, oils, and countless other chemically induced ingredients.

Sugar: Sugar is a simple crystalline carbohydrate taken most often from sugar cane and sugar beet to sweeten foods and drinks. Added sugar is found in just about all food products we buy today and huge amounts can be found in the sodas and juices we buy as well. This little added ingredient is everywhere! The thing that is important to understand is this tiny, sweet additive is one of the worst ingredients added to our foods and drinks today. The amount we consume is toxic! Our children live on sugar and eat far too much of this ingredient on a daily and consistent basis. We are setting them up to face huge health issues in the future. Research is suggesting and pointing us in the direction that sugar is absolutely contributing to many of the diseases and conditions we are facing. How can sugar be that bad for us? Let's get right to the point:

- Sugar is addictive and creates acidity in the body. It is a huge problem for someone with Candida. It creates that vicious, vicious cycle I talked about earlier that make us crave sugary foods and drinks. We crave sugar because the yeast needs it in order to survive and multiply.
- Sugar can damage your heart by affecting the pumping mechanism which may increase risk of heart failure. It has also been associated with dyslipidemia which increases the risk of heart disease.
- Sugar promotes belly fat (your body has to store it somewhere).
- Sugar is linked to cancer production and free radical initiators.
- Sugar has the same effect on the body as alcohol. A sugar addiction can lead to an alcohol addiction. The health effects caused by drinking too much alcohol are the same for someone who consumes too much sugar.
- Sugar has been found to have a positive correlation to the aging of our cells.
- Sugar has been linked to diabetes.

- Sugar has been linked to obesity. Obesity has been linked to heart disease, kidney disease, and diabetes.
- Sugar is linked to increased blood pressure.
- Sugar is linked to changes in metabolism.
- Sugar can suppress the immune system.
- Sugar causes hyperactivity and anxiety in children. It can increase the risk of school related learning problems.
- Sugar causes copper and chromium deficiencies.
- Sugar interferes with the body's ability to absorb calcium, magnesium, and proteins.
- Sugar can impair the structure of DNA and reduce high-density lipoproteins and growth hormones.
- Sugar increases the risk of or can aggravate Crohn's disease, colitis, ulcers, arthritis, hemorrhoids, varicose veins, gallstones, periodontal disease, osteoporosis, food allergies, eczema, cataracts, emphysema, asthma, migraine headaches, irritable bowel syndrome, and acne.
- Sugar causes inflammation, fatigue, moodiness, headaches, weakened eyesight, heart palpitations, muscle pains, and tremors.

Basically, sugar adds stress to the body and over time leads to a toxic build up which we know leaves us in a state of acidity. We also know that a state of acidity leads to inflammation which leads to symptoms, illnesses, and eventually disease.

We don't have to be in fear of sugar. I am not asking you to avoid it always and forever. That is one hundred percent impossible. We just have to begin to recognize how much of it we are consuming on a daily basis. We can begin to take back control of our bodies and demand better from the companies who are producing foods with this ingredient.

Soy: Soy, and products that contain soy, is another area of the food maze to be aware of as this ingredient is found in a wide variety of packaged and processed foods. From 2000-2007, U.S. food manufacturers introduced more than 2,700 new soy-based foods. From 1995-2012, the U.S. government subsidized this industry with $27.8 billion of taxpayer monies. Soy is a type of bean. Soy derivatives can now be found in soups, mayonnaise, salad dressings, cookies, margarine, fast food, baking mixes, infant formula, tofu, vegetarian "meats", cereal, candy, sauces and gravies, frozen food, vitamins, deli meats, Asian foods, chocolate, energy bars, and vegetable and chicken broths.

People in this country began eating soy in larger quantities as a result of the soybean industry's massive marketing campaign touting the benefits of soy. As more studies have come out about this product, there is growing controversy concerning its health benefits to us. My understanding is the health benefits and risks of soy depend solely on whether or not the soy has been properly fermented.

Fermentation is an aging process in which the soy protein is broken down into smaller chains or into single amino acids. These smaller chains or amino acids aid in digestion and reduce potential allergic reactions. Properly fermented soy can lower cholesterol and is high in protein and fiber. This process also increases the absorption of vital nutrients due to the beneficial bacteria. It is important that the soy you consume has been through the proper fermentation process. This necessary process kills the toxins on the bean before consumption. Most of the soy sold and consumed today has not been through the proper fermentation process and poses a potential health risk. You won't hear the soy industry warning you of this difference. Unfermented soy (what we typically eat today) has been associated with food allergies, digestive disorders, immune-system breakdown, thyroid problems, cancer, infertility, malnutrition, heart disease, ADD, ADHD, and PMS symptoms. Not only is most of the soy grown in the United States not fermented properly, a large percentage of this crop is now genetically modified. The impact this ingredient has on the human body over a long period of time (decades) and the amount now being consumed in its unfermented state is a cause for concern for all of us.

Examples of healthy fermented soy include: tempeh, natto, miso, pickled tofu, tamari (fermented soy sauce), and fermented tofu. Edamame has not been through the fermentation process. For anyone who is questioning if they suffer from Candida related symptoms, fermented food is not a good option. Tofu and edamame in general are a healthier option than foods that have been processed with soy derivatives because they have not been heavily processed.

The ingredients listed below are also soy derivatives:

- Hydrolyzed protein
- MSG
- Soy lecithin
- Soy protein
- Soybean oil
- Teriyaki sauce
- Textured vegetable protein
- Artificial flavoring
- Plant protein
- Vegetable broth, gum, and starch

Gluten: What is gluten and why is it important to understand? Going on a gluten-free diet seems to be one of the latest diet crazes or nutritional fads today. Gluten is a protein found in products containing wheat, rye, and barley. Wheat Subsidies in the United States totaled $35.5 billion from 1995-2012.

A huge amount of processed foods and baked goods contain wheat. It is fair to say the consumer is ingesting a large amount of gluten each day for their entire life. It can typically be found in breads, cookies, grains, pastries, bagels, donuts, crackers, muffins, pasta noodles, and more. It is used for the purposes of enhancing taste and texture, as a thickening agent, and can be used as a source of protein. Gluten derivatives can also now be discovered in salad dressing, cereal, broths, gravies, sauces, vitamins, toothpaste, and some prescription medications.

Gluten's use in diverse foods and condiments is increasing. The amount of gluten now being digested in our diet today far surpasses that of our ancestors just a few generations ago. One of the concerns is that gluten causes inflammation and triggers or increases the body's immune system response. Our bodies are reacting to this negatively enhanced protein because our body is not equipped to digest the amount now being consumed. On top of that, the wheat we eat today is now being genetically modified to contain increased amounts of gluten. We are consuming more gluten because it has been genetically altered and because it can be found in more and more food products as a "filler" ingredient. Just as our digestive system has trouble digesting corn and soy, the same can be said for gluten. It can cause intestinal irritation and damage the small intestine. The small intestine's functions as a catalyst for absorbing the nutrients we eat and drink on a daily basis. Gluten has the ability to increase inflammation and adversely affect autoimmune diseases. Gluten sensitivities can be linked to fatigue, anemia, bloating, abdominal pain, leaky gut syndrome, depression, headaches, brain function, eczema, joint pain, and contributes to cancer growth. The body's ability to properly absorb essential nutrients by the way of the small intestine can be compromised with gluten sensitivities. We are all sensitive to the amount of gluten being consumed today.

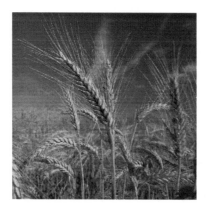

The food industry's desire to financially profit from the increasing consumer demand for gluten-free foods is growing. In 2012, the U.S. Department of Agriculture estimated the gluten-free industry will reach $1.9 billion in revenue. It can be a challenge to find gluten-free foods that are "healthy" and within your budget. Be aware that just because a product says that it is gluten-free does not necessarily mean it is packed with nutrients or that it is good for us.

By reading the ingredients on the packaging of products you will discover that cornmeal and corn flour, rice flour, potato flour, millet flour, amaranth flour, tapioca flour, and arrowroot flour are all popular alternatives to the other flours containing gluten.

It was a process for me to decrease gluten from my diet. I began by eliminating foods such as pasta, breads, cereals, crackers, and baked goods.

Recommendations for you or your family:

- Increase your intake of fruits, vegetables, nuts, seeds, and beans.
- Reduce processed or packaged foods
- Brown rice and quinoa are also good alternatives.
- Gluten-free flours include: amaranth, arrowroot, white and brown rice flour, buckwheat, millet, tapioca, and sorghum flour.
- Simply reduce the amount of baked goods and bread your family is consuming.
- There are a few brands to look for while shopping that can help you transition to a reduction in your gluten intake. These brands include products such as: breads, cookies, pasta, pie and pizza crusts, bagels, rolls, buns, tortillas, muffins, and cake and brownie mixes. Gluten-free brands include: Udi's (www.udisglutenfree.com), Glutino (www.glutino.com), Annie's (www.annies.com), Hol-Grain (www.hol-grain.com), Bob's (www.bobsredmill.com), and Schar (www.schar.com) These are all popular brands and can be found in most grocery stores.

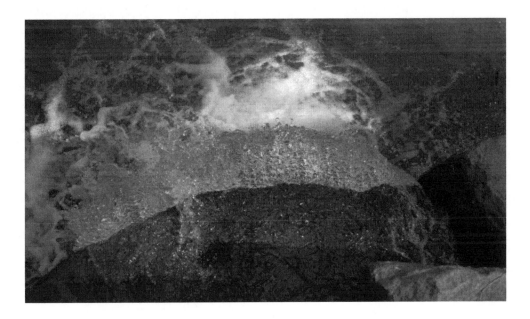

Water: The consumption of water is vital to our overall health and well-being. All living things must have access to it in order to survive. The United States has one of the "safest" water supplies in the world. We are fortunate that water is freely available to most people. We rarely have to consider where our water comes from in this country. We have developed a process of purifying water that eradicates most potentially harmful organisms to our bodies.

Water makes up over half of our body weight and over seventy percent of the world's surface areas. It is a chemical compound often referred to as H_2O. It is made up of one part oxygen atom and two parts hydrogen atoms.

Proper hydration contributes too many positive health benefits. Some of the health benefits of drinking water include: weight loss, energizing of muscles, keeps skin looking healthy, helps to maintain normal body functions, assists the kidneys in flushing out toxins, reduces fluid retention, helps to maintain normal bowel function, boosts the immune system, increases energy, decreases fatigue, and balances the body's fluids. It can help in the digestion, absorption, circulation, and transportation of nutrients throughout the body. Water is an absolute necessity for our bodies.

Let's consider for a moment the problems associated with our current water supply and the negative, cumulative effects additives and toxins can potentially have on our health.

The water that we have direct access to in our homes is controlled by local governments or municipalities. It is their responsibility to maintain the water treatment centers in your area and to ensure the public has adequate and safe drinking water. To do this effectively, it has been decided for you that chemicals will be added to the water supply. The problem is that, yet again, we do not fully understand the ramifications of such decisions on our health. An ABC News study revealed there are over 700 chemicals in our drinking water and 129 of those chemicals have been tested by the EPA as potentially causing serious health risks and problems. The two most widely known chemicals deliberately added to our water are chlorine and fluoride.

Chlorine is added to kill off bugs. The problem is chlorine is a free radical initiator, potentially elevating cholesterol levels and accelerating the aging process. Your body takes in more chlorine through your skin than it does drinking eight glasses of water a day. Fluoride is added to our water supply for the sole purpose of supposedly strengthening our teeth and decreasing tooth decay. This chemical does not improve the quality of the water or kill off bugs or microorganisms. The problem with fluoride is it damages important enzymes (including in the brain), causes cellular dysfunction, damages hormone receptors, and can cause excessive calcification in arteries, joints, and ligaments.

We also need to be aware of other contaminants that dirty our water supply including the run-off of fertilizers and pesticides from agriculture. Heavy metals such as mercury, lead, and cadmium also contaminate the water supply. Petrochemical products such as gasoline, diesel, and benzene can contaminate the water from underground storage tanks. Dioxins, prescriptions medications, arsenic, radioactive materials, PCB's, and medical waste are still other examples of toxins that have found their way into our water supply as a result of industrial waste and an attitude that is indifferent to the poisoning of a precious resource. We should ALL care! What are we leaving our children? The health risks associated to our children from these chemicals that we dump into the water supply also include: cellular dysfunction, damage to the endocrine and immune system, brain abnormalities, fatigue, lower blood cell functioning, the ability to carry oxygen to all of the body, muscle aches, different types of cancer, neurotoxicity, Candida infection, damage to the kidneys, joints, and reproductive system, bone disease, skin disease, liver damage, and anemia to name a few.

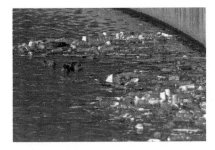 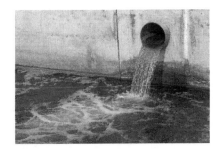

While it is important to drink plenty of water each day, it is equally important to find a clean source of water.

Different types of purification systems for you to consider and research that decrease contaminants include:

- Distilled water
- Reverse osmosis
- Ultraviolet disinfection
- Commercial filters
- Structured water
- Ionization process

In the last few years I have used distilled, filtered, and reverse osmosis water for my family. You can go to www.foodandwaterwatch.org/take-action/consumer-tools/choosing-a-water-filter to learn more.

Fast Food: Everything a fast food restaurant does from marketing, advertising, and product labeling, to the inclusion of toys in its children's meals and choosing a restaurant location is one hundred percent geared to get our children consuming this food now and for a lifetime. It is a vast business empire with the health of our children on the line.

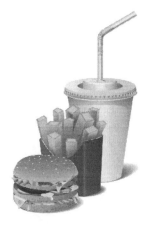

Here is what I consider to be some of the main problems associated with fast food:

- It is factory-style food. When you are producing a product in vast quantities, the nutritional value or quality of the food declines. The beef and chicken are all grown on factory farms and all of the fruits and vegetables are grown on commercial farms. Pesticides, fertilizers, genetic modification, antibiotics, steroids, and growth hormones are all part of your meal in some combination.

- Fast food is loaded with sugars, salts, preservatives, and fatty oils.

- The kitchens of all fast-food restaurants are mini factories in terms of preparation from beginning to end. The goal is to have the food appear exactly the same and to get you in and out as quickly as possible.

- We now have a generation of children who are regularly eating fast food in place of home cooked meals. This generation has a huge obesity problem that will lead to significant health problems in the future including high cholesterol, high blood pressure, and heart disease.

- The burgers are now filled with meat fillers. Meat fillers are unwanted meat parts at the time of slaughter that are processed and made into a paste. This paste is added to ground beef to give the appearance of a big, juicy burger. This beef filler product is becoming hugely popular for fast food chains as they analyze ways to increase profit and minimize costs. During the process of making paste, ammonia is added to kill off pathogens. This supposedly makes the beef safer from microorganisms. It is cheap to make and saves fast food companies pennies on every pound of ground beef.

- Fast food is missing most nutrients, vitamins, and minerals that children need to sustain a growing body.

- Another hidden danger lies in the very product used to wrap our fast-food burgers and sandwiches, the wrapper. A new study shows that the toxin, perfluoroalkyl or perfluoroalkyl substances (PFASs), which is used in surface protection treatments and coatings to keep grease from leaking through fast food wrappers, is being ingested by people. As a result, this contaminant is showing up in their blood. Perfluoroalkyls are a hazardous class of stable, synthetic chemicals that repel oil, grease, and water. These chemicals have been linked to: infertility, thyroid disease, cancer, immune-system problems, and increased LDL cholesterol levels.

- In 2008, a study was conducted on eight different brands of fast-food hamburgers. The purpose of the study was to scientifically study, analyze, evaluate, and determine the content of the hamburgers. The results were extensive. What I found most interesting is that in seven of the eight brands tested, more than twenty fragments of skeletal muscle, connective tissue, and blood vessels were noted in all hamburgers.

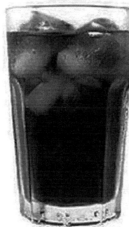

7 Side Effects of Soda

Phosphoric Acid - Weakens bones and rots teeth

Excessive artificial sweeteners makes you crave more

Carmel Color - Made from the chemical caramel, is purely cosmetic, it doesn't add flavor yet is tainted with carcinogens.

Formaldehyde - Carcinogen, it is not added in soda but when you digest aspartame, it will break down into 2 amino acids and methanol = formic acid + formaldehyde (diet sodas)

High Fructose Corn Syrup is a Concentrated form of sugar, fructose derived from corn. It increases body fat, cholesterol and triglycerides and it also makes you hungry.

Potassium Benzoate = preservative that can be broken down to benzene in your body. Keep your soda in the sun and benzene = Carcinogen

Food Dyes = impaired brain function, hyperactive behavior, difficulty focussing, lack of impulse control.

Dave Sommers

Interesting Statistics on Fast Food:

- In 1970, Americans spent about $6 billion on fast food. In 2006, the spending rose to nearly $142 billion.
- There are more than 300,000 fast food restaurants in the U.S. alone.
- Television has greatly expanded the ability of advertisers to reach children in an attempt to develop brand loyalty early in life. Today, the average American child sees more than 10,000 food advertisements each year on television.
- Eating fast food can result in high levels of insulin which has been linked to rising incidences of type 2 diabetes.
- Dangerous fast food ingredients have been linked to various cancers and obesity including: MSG, trans fat, sodium nitrite, BHA, BHT, Propyl gallate, aspartame, acesulfame-K, olestra, potassium bromate, and food coloring: Blue 1 and 2; Red 3; Green 3; and Yellow 6.
- The average distance from a fast food restaurant in the U.S. to a school is half a mile.
- The U.S. fast-food industry serves more than 50 million Americans each and every day.
- Half of the average American's yearly food budget is spent at fast-food chains.
- In the 1950's, a typical fast food hamburger wighed one ounce. Today, a hamburger now weigh six ounces.
- The Federal Trade Commission (FTC) reports the U.S. fast-food industry spends approximately $1.6 billion each year on marketing aimed at children.
- Americans spend more money per year on fast food than they do on education.

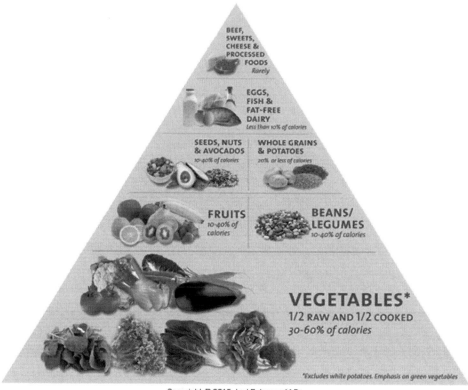

Copyright © 2010 Joel Fuhrman M.D.

Now consider this food pyramid after reading about the dangers of our current food supply. What can you change or implement into your daily eating habits? Visit www.drfuhrman.com for more information and resources. You can also read his informative book, <u>Eat To Live</u>.

References

1. Environmental Protection Agency, Crop Production, Accessed on May 20, 2011, http://www.epa.gov/agriculture/ag101/printcrop.html

2. Environmental Working Group, Corn Subsidies, Accessed on July 14, 2011, http://farm.ewg.org/progdetail.php?fips=00000&progcode=corn

3. Livestrong.com, "Health Risks of High Fructose Corn Syrup", Accessed on August 4, 2011, http://www.livestrong.com/article/259181-health-risks-of-high-fructose-corn-syrup/

4. Global Healing Center, 5 Health Dangers of High Fructose Corn Syrup, Accessed on My 7, 2014, http://www.globalhealingcenter.com/natural-health/high-fructose-corn-syrup-dangers/

5. USA TODAY, "Study: fructose corn syrup contains mercury", Accessed on November 18, 2010, http://www.usatoday.com/news/health/2009-01-27-corn-syrup_N.htm

6. Huffington Post, "The Not-So-Sweet Truth About High Fructose Corn Syrup", Accessed on May 17, 2011, http://www.huffingtonpost.com/dr-mark-hyman/high-fructose-corn-syrup-dangers_b_86193.html

7. Princeton University, "A sweet problem: Princeton researchers find that high-fructose corn syrup prompts considerably more weight gain", Accessed on May 7, 2014, http://www.princeton.edu/main/news//archive/S26/91/22K07/

8. The American Journal of Clinical Nutrition, "Consumption of high fructose corn syrup in beverages may play a role in the epidemic of obesity", Accessed on May 7, 2014, http:/ajcn.nutrition.org/content/79/4/537.full

9. "corn-derived food ingredients I avoid", Accessed on May 17, 2011. http://www.vishniac.com/ephrain/corn-brother.html

10. Live Corn Free, "Ingredients Derived From Corn – What to Avoid", Accessed on May 17, 2011, http"//www.livecornfree.com/2010/04/ingredients-derived-from-corn-what-to.html

11. Environmental Working Group, Soybean Subsidies, Accessed on May 8, 2014, http://www.farm.ewg.org/progdetail.php?fips=00000&progcode=soybean

12. About.com, "List of Soy Ingredients to Avoid when Following a Soy-Free Diet", Accessed on October, 30, 2013, http://foodallergies.about.com/od/soyallergies/a/List-Of-Soy-Ingredietns-To-Avoid-When-Following-A-Soy-Free-Diet.htm

13. Talk About Curing Autism (TACA), What is Soy, Accessed on May 8, 2014, http://www.tacanow.org/family-resources/what-is-soy/

14. Mercola.com, "Soy: This "Miracle Health Food" Has Been Linked to Brain Damage and Breast Cancer", Accessed on May 8, 2014, http://articles.mercola.com/sites/articles/archive/2010/09/18/soy-can-damage-your-health.aspx

15. Essential Formulas.com, The Benefits of Soy Fermentation, Accessed on May 8, 2014, http://www.essentialformulas.com/efi.cgim?template=information_on_soy_fermentation

16. Natural News, "Fermented Soy is Only Soy Food Fit for Human Consumption", Accessed on May 8, 2014, http://www.naturalnews.com/025513_soy_food_soybeans.html

17. Livestrong.com, "Why is Gluten Bad For Me", Accessed on October 1, 2012, http://www.livestrong.com/articleg/422103-why-is-gluten-bad-for-me/

18. Statistic Brain, Gluten/Celiac Disease Statistics, Accessed on May 8, 2014, http"//www.statisticbrain.com/gluten-celiac-disease-statistics/

19. Chronic fatigue and nutrition.com, "What's The Problem With Gluten", Accessed on May 8, 2014, http://chronicfatigueandnutrition.com/gluten-problem/what%e2%80%99s-the-problem-with-gluten/

20. Environmental Working Group, Wheat Subsidies, Accessed on May 8, 2014, http://farm.ewg.org/progdetail.php?fips=00000&progcode=wheat

21. The Environment Illness Resource, Common Chemical Contaminants of Water, Accessed on November 10, 2013, http://www.ei-resource.org/common-chemical-contaminants-of-municipal-water/

22. Inorganic Elements in Tap Water, Accessed on August 2, 2011, http://www.chem.duke.edu/~jds/cruise_chem/water/watinorg.html

23. Realfoods.net, What's Wrong with Tap Water, Accessed on August 2, 2011, http://www.realfoods.net/tapwater.html

24. Huffington Post, "What is in Fast Food? A newly Discovered Reason to Avoid Fast Food", Accessed on December 20, 2010, http://www.huffingtonpost.com/dr-mercola/fast-food-health_b_800297.htm

25. Science Direct, "Fast food hamburgers: What are we really eating?" Accessed on August 3, 2011, available online at http://www. sciencedirect.com/science/article/pii/S1092913408000622

26. Random Facts, 55 Juicy Facts about Fast Food, accessed on August 3, 2011, http://facts.randomhistory.com/2009/06/27_fast-food.html

27. Fatburn-Secrets.com, Scary Fast Food Statistics & Facts, Accessed on August 3, 2011, http://www.fatburn-secrets.com/fast-food-statistics.html

CHAPTER 10
The So-Called Healthy Foods: Fruits and Vegetables

"It's an unsustainable system that relies heavily on chemical fertilizers...to keep yields high and produce 'hollow food.'"

—KEN WARREN

Ideally fruits and vegetables provide many nutrients to our bodies when consumed. The larger the quantity of these foods eaten, the more nutrients we will take in. Fruits and vegetables provide us with natural, earthly forms of fiber, zinc, vitamin C, iron, calcium, phosphorous, vitamin A, potassium, manganese, vitamin K, protein, pectin, copper, selenium, vitamin E, folic acid, and antioxidants. These nutrients inhibit cancer growth, regulate blood sugar, lower cholesterol, aid in digestion, relieve joint pain, lower cardiovascular diseases, fight inflammation, relieve arthritis symptoms, aid in weight loss, increase functioning of nervous and immune system, help with depression and infertility, improve eyesight, prevent a host of diseases, and increase energy levels.

According to the U.S. Census Bureau, there are roughly 318 million people currently living in the Unites States. If everyone is directed to eat several servings of fruits and vegetables a day, how can we grow that many crops each and every day to sustain the demand? I would say innovative technology in farming techniques and machinery throughout the last century has helped to meet the growing demand. We can now grow crops faster, in larger quantities, and all-year round. However, there are three main points that I wish to share with you concerning the harvesting and production of this country's fruits and vegetables.

Pesticides are chemicals used to eliminate or control a variety of agricultural pests that damage crops and livestock and reduce farm productivity. The most commonly applied pesticides are: insecticides (to kill insects), herbicides (to kill weeds), rodenticides (to kill rodents), and fungicides (to kill fungi, mold, and mildew).

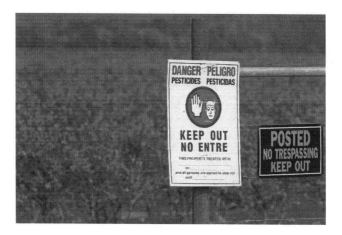

Over 1 billion tons of pesticides are used in the United States every year. There are 20,000 different pesticides now registered with the Environmental Protection Agency. These pesticides can also be directly sprayed on cattle to ward off flies, spiders, and other insects found in the grain (corn) the cattle consume.

Pesticides are a public health concern and have been linked to a range of diseases and disorders. Many chemical pesticides are known to cause poisoning, infertility, birth defects, damage to the nervous system, and may potentially cause cancer. A study conducted by the Canadian government concluded that chemical pesticides might contribute to testicular, brain, prostate, breast, and stomach cancer. We spray or apply pesticides on the outside of fruits and vegetables during the course of the growth cycle. As a result, the pesticide residue is consumed by all of us.

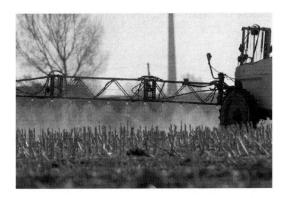 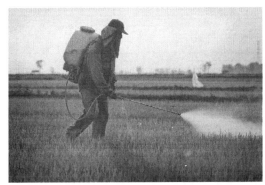

Below is a list of fruits and vegetables that have been compiled by the Environmental Working Group listing the highest pesticide residue based on USDA and FDA testing data for 2015. This list is compiled on a yearly basis.

If you consume these products, please take advantage of the opportunity to buy organic or you may want to consider not buying them at all.

- Apples
- Peaches
- Sweet bell peppers
- Celery
- Nectarines (imported)
- Strawberries
- Grapes
- Spinach
- Cherry tomatoes

- Cucumbers
- Potatoes
- Snap peas

Below are fruits and vegetables that have lower pesticide residue according to The Environmental Working Group for 2015.

- Onion
- Avocado
- Mango
- Asparagus
- sweet peas
- kiwi
- cabbage
- eggplant
- papaya
- Sweet corn
- sweet potato
- cauliflower
- cantaloupe
- grapefruit
- pineapple

According to the Environmental Working Group, consumers can reduce their pesticide exposure by 80 percent by avoiding the most contaminated produce. The produce above has lower pesticide residue because either the outer layer protects the actual food or because these crops do not need as much protection from insects and weeds. Thus, they require a more limited pesticide management program.

2. Chemical Fertilizers are chemical compounds applied to the soil underneath and around crops to promote growth. Fertilizers provide direct nutrients to the soil that have been depleted and overused year after year. I want to talk with you about chemical fertilizers and what you may not know about the hidden dangers. Most agricultural and commercial farms use chemicals and hazardous waste to fertilize the fruits and vegetables we are purchasing in all grocery stores around this country. I am also referring to the fertilizers that you buy at your local nursery or hardware store to use on your own lawn or garden.

The fertilizer industry is a $60 billion dollar a year entity. Chemical fertilizers contain three main ingredients. These ingredients are nitrogen, phosphorus, and potassium. Other nutrients can be included in fertilizers to further enhance or vitalize the richness of the soil. Examples might include calcium, magnesium, and iron. However, there are many causes of concern when it comes to the use of chemical fertilizers being used to nourish the soil our fruits and vegetables are grown in. While calcium, magnesium, and iron are added nutrients used to enhance soil vitality, it is the hidden danger, hazardous waste and its' bi-products, included in with these ingredients that pose the danger. I wish this issue was as simple as saying the soil is being depleted of essential nutrients, we need to find ways to bring back into balance the depletion of the soil's vital nutrients, and that enhancing the ground with fertilizers is a viable and healthy option for us.

Large corporations and small businesses alike have found and take advantage of loopholes in government regulations in regard to the disposal of hazardous waste.

The Environmental Protection Agency (EPA) is an agency of the federal government charged with protecting human health and the environment by writing and enforcing laws and regulations. In 2013, the EPA employed over 17,000 people at a cost to taxpayers of $8.2 billion dollars. The EPA states hazardous waste is waste that is dangerous or potentially harmful to our health or the environment.

Hazardous wastes can be liquids, solids, gases, or sludge's. This waste can be flammable, reactive (can explode), corrosive, and toxic. They can be discarded commercial products such as cleaning fluids and pesticides or the bi-product of the manufacturing process. Dry cleaners, print shops, automobile repair centers, oil refineries, and pest control companies are examples of companies that produce hazardous waste.

The shipment of hazardous waste to the proper disposal site is extremely expensive and cuts down on the profit of a company producing hazardous waste. Unfortunately, companies have figured out a way to get rid of their hazardous waste in a very cost effective manner. **They are recycling their hazardous waste and**

toxins into chemical fertilizer for commercial farming and home gardening! I will say it again because it is important for you to understand. **Companies are now recycling their EPA classified hazardous waste and toxins into chemical fertilizer for commercial farming and home gardening.**

According to the article, *Killing Fields? Toxic waste Being Spread as Fertilizer* by Duff Wilson, manufacturing industries are disposing of hazardous waste materials by turning them into fertilizers to spread across farms all over this country. What we are not being told is this toxic waste contains plutonium (isn't that used in making nuclear bombs?), arsenic, mercury, cadmium, and lead among many other toxins. Another potential chemical included in chemical fertilizers is dioxin. Dioxin is the most dangerous chemical known to science.

Tests conducted by the state of Washington have concluded that some fertilizers contained one hundred times higher the level allowed for treated superfund sites in that state. According to *Voice of the Environment,* one recent study discovered twenty-two heavy metals in all twenty-nine fertilizers tested. Many of these contaminants are known to cause cancer, reproductive and developmental toxicity, or other serious health effects in varying degrees. 100 percent of the children in the U.S. are known to have received toxic exposure to neurotoxic substances above the U.S. government health guidelines. The *Voice of the Environment* also states recent studies show that between 1990 and 1995, 600 companies from 44 states sent 270 million pounds of toxic waste to farms and fertilizer companies across the country. This waste included 69 different types of toxins including 13.9 million pounds of known carcinogens.

An article dating back to 2003 states 110 billion pounds of commercial fertilizer and 4.2 million pounds of sewage sludge were spread across American farmlands, public spaces, and home gardens. There has been no federal requirement that toxins be listed as ingredients on fertilizer labels and there is no testing of these substances or compounds on human health. There are federal laws that outline regulations to chemical fertilizer's manufacturing, distribution, and use. However, the Environmental Protection Agency does not want to regulate the fertilizer industry. It is up to the states to regulate this industry. As I began my research a few years ago on this topic, only four states had begun to address this issue. The production of chemical fertilizers from hazardous waste, by companies wanting to save money regardless of the environmental and human health impact, is one of the greatest examples I have found yet of corporate greed and governmental indifference.

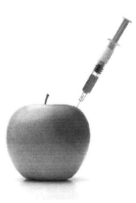

3. **Genetically modified Organisms (GMO's)** are becoming more and more common today as scientists and biotech companies look for ways to produce large quantities of fruits and vegetables to sustain a growing population. Genetically modified organisms are typically plant based foods derived from genetically altered organisms. Genetically modified organisms have had specific changes introduced into their DNA by genetic engineering techniques. Genetic modification is a method used by scientists in a laboratory to introduce new traits or characteristics to an organism. The biotech companies, with acceptance from the food industry and our government, are altering the fruits and vegetables we eat by changing their genetic make-up. We are told they are doing this for several reasons:

- To develop techniques to grow more food and quickly
- To increase the nutritional value of a specific crop
- To develop strategies to limit crop damage from exposure to insects and weeds
- To increase the ripeness and taste of a fruit or vegetable

It is fair to say that GMO crops are now herbicide, pesticide, and supposedly disease resistant. They will be less adversely affected by the natural elements during their life cycle and growing season.

The problem is there are many flaws and areas of concern in this process. There are on-going debates as to whether GMO's are safe for human consumption. The biggest health threat to humans is that no one knows how this will affect our long-term health. This potential health threat also includes the ethical responsibility of the biotech companies (they might actually have all the data as it pertains to the dangers posed to us and have decided we do not need to know), the food industry, the government, and the medical community at large. No one knows the true impact on our health in the long run because GMO foods have only been around since the 1990's.

The environmental concerns of GMO crops are widespread. They include unintended harm to other organisms, reduced effectiveness of pesticides, and gene transfer to non-target species. One of the biggest concerns today surrounding GMO food on the human body is it increases allergic reactions which can lead to a whole host of health issues that accumulate over a lifetime. If allergies are increasing in our children at an accelerated rate, is it possible that GMO food is part of the problem? While there is limited scientific research regarding GMO foods on human health, in 2009 The American Academy of Environmental Medicine (AAEM) stated that several animal studies indicate serious health risks associated with GMO food including: infertility, immune problems, accelerated aging, and changes in major organs. According to the Organic Consumers Association, GMO food can create unpredictable and hard to detect side effects such as infertility, allergies, toxins, cell growth (precursor to cancer), infant mortality, new diseases and nutritional problems.

According to the Non-GMO Project, the following list is at-risk crops for genetic modification:
- Alfalfa
- Canola
- Corn
- Cotton
- Papaya
- Soy
- Sugar Beets
- Zucchini and yellow summer squash

According to the Non-GMO Project, the following list is monitored crops for genetic modification:

- Chard, table beets
- Rutabaga, Siberian kale
- Bok Choy, Chinese cabbage, turnip
- Acorn squash
- Flax
- Rice
- Wheat

In 1994, tomatoes became the first commercially produced GMO. In 1997, they were brought out of production due to problems with flavor and shelf-life. Genetically modified potatoes were introduced in 1996. This product was stopped in 2001 due to rejection by the public.

Most developed nations do not consider GMO's to be safe. More than 60 countries including Australia, Japan, and all countries in the European Union have significant restrictions or bans in place regarding this practice. In the United States, the government has approved GMO's based on studies by the same corporations that create and profit from them.

Crops are now being genetically altered or modified to resist the spraying of these certain pesticides. On June 7th, 2011, a report called, *"Roundup and birth defects: Is the public being kept in the Dark?"* became public. The article states regulators knew as far back as 1980 that glyphosate, the chemical on which Roundup is based, can cause birth defects in laboratory animals. The report comes months after researchers found that genetically modified crops, used in conjunction with Roundup, contain a pathogen that may cause animal miscarriages. This pesticide will not be government reviewed with more stringent, up-to-date standards until 2030.

The largest producer of genetically modified crops and seeds is a company called Monsanto that I discussed earlier. Monsanto was founded in 1901 as a chemical company. The company's first product was the artificial sweetener, saccharin. It also introduced caffeine and vanillin to Coca Cola and became one of that company's main suppliers. By 1920, the company expanded its operations to include basic industrial chemicals. By the 1940's, it was a leading manufacturer of plastics. It has remained one of the top ten U.S. chemical companies. It has also been responsible for the introduction of specific herbicides, DDT, Agent Orange, the artificial sweetener aspartame, PCB's, and the bovine growth hormone (rBGH).

Monsanto scientists became the first to genetically modify a plant cell in 1982. Five years later, Monsanto conducted the first field tests of genetically engineered crops. From 1997-2002, Monsanto made a transition from a chemical giant to a biotech giant. Monsanto is responsible for the substantial increase in genetically modified seeds as well as the controversial pesticide, Roundup. Monsanto has scientifically engineered the genetic alteration of specific seeds to withstand the spraying of this pesticide. The seeds are able to resist the pesticide being sprayed on more and more conventional crops. The farmers spray the crops, the weeds or insects die, but the crop is still viable. You are left with a fruit or vegetable that contains a pesticide on the outside and a different genetic makeup on the inside. It is important to understand that Monsanto holds the power in regard to the safety and viability of seeds all over the world.

Below are some of the problems you need to be aware of concerning Monsanto and genetically modified crops. This is important because it directly and personally affects you and your family's health and longevity:

- In 1998, Phil Angell, who was the director of Corporate Communications for Monsanto stated, "Monsanto should not have to vouchsafe the safety of biotech food. Our interest is in selling as much of it as possible. Assuring its safety is the FDA's job."

- A huge conflict of interest is occurring between Monsanto and the very people we elect to work on our behalf. Take a look at the individuals who have worked for Monsanto and for government agencies that oversee our nation's food supply including regulation and safety. I would conclude we are the ones who will unknowingly pay for this conflict of interest, if we aren't already.

Person	Government Job	Monsanto Job
Clarence Thomas (R)	U.S. Supreme Court Justice	Former Monsanto lawyer
Michael Taylor (D)	FDA Deputy Commissioner for Foods	Former Monsanto Vice President
Ann Veneman	Secretary of Agriculture	BOD-Monsanto Calgene Corporation
Linda Fisher	Deputy Administrator of the EPA	Head of Governmental Affairs for Monsanto
Michael Friedman	Commissioner of the FDA	Senior VP for Clinical Affairs at G.D. Searle & Co. (a pharmaceutical division of Monsanto)
William Ruckelshaus	Chief Administrator of the EPA	BOD-Monsanto
Mickey Kantor	Secretary of Commerce	BOD-Monsanto
Donald Rumsfeld (R)	Secretary of Defense	BOD-Monsanto's Searle Pharmaceuticals
Tommy Thompson (D)	U.S. Secretary of Health	Received $50,000 in donations from Monsanto during Wisconsin's governor's race
John Ashcroft (R)	U.S. Attorney General	Received monetary donation from Monsanto during run for office
Larry Combest	Chairman of the House Agricultural Committee	Received money from Monsanto while running for office
Carol Tucker Foreman	"consumer advocate" on U.S. Biotech Consultative Forum Delegation	Monsanto Lobbyist

Person	Government Job	Monsanto Job
Marcia Hale	Assistant to the President of the United States	Director of International Affairs for Monsanto
Josh King	Director of Production White House Events	Director of Global Communication for Monsanto
Tom Vilsack (D)	USDA Secretary	Pro-biotech former governor of Iowa
Roger Beachy (D)	USDA National Institute of Food and Agriculture	Former director of the Monsanto funded Danforth Plant Science Center
Islam Siddiqui (D)	Agriculture Negotiator for the U.S. Trade Representative	Former VP of the Monsanto and Dupont lobbying group CropLife (promoted pesticides)
Rajiv Shah (D)	USDA Under Secretary for Research and Education and Economics. Current head of USAID	Former Agricultural Development director for the pro-biotech Gates Foundation (a frequent Monsanto partner)
Elena Kagan (D)	U.S. Supreme Court Justice	As solicitor general, she took Monsanto's side against organic farmers in the Round-Up Ready alfalfa court case
Margaret Miller (D)	FDA Official	Former Monsanto Researcher

(R)-Republican (D)-Democrat (BOD) - Board of Directors Member

- An anonymous document in 2001 identified Monsanto as being a potential responsible party in fifty-six contaminated Superfund sites in the United States. A Superfund site is abandoned properly where hazardous material is discarded. Monsanto has been sued and has settled multiple times for damaging the health of its employees or residents near these sites.
- Monsanto is the largest producer of glyphosate herbicides through its popular brand, Roundup. While using Roundup ready seeds offer a convenient method for farmers to kill insects, parasites, and weeds, studies suggest that this ingredient is toxic.
- Farmers have saved their seeds from season to season for centuries. Monsanto is now developing and patenting seeds that can no longer be used from season to season. Their lifecycle is one season. Farmers will have to purchase seeds every year. Historically, the United States Patent and Trademark Office had refused to grant patents on seeds considering them a life source with too many variables. In 1980, the Unites States Supreme Court ruled against this line of thinking. This opened up the ability to patent seeds. Monsanto has since become the world leader in the genetic modification of seeds. It has obtained 674 biotechnology patents.
- Monsanto is acquiring and will one day have the ability to possibly control the world's seed supply. In 2005, Monsanto purchased a company that owned 40 percent of the U.S. market for lettuce, tomatoes, and other vegetable and fruit seeds. It is estimated that Monsanto seeds now account for 90 percent of the U.S. production of soybeans. One school of thought is that whoever controls the world's seeds supply, will one day control the world's food supply. Do we really want one company to control the world's seed supply?
- In 1980, no genetically modified crops were grown in the United States. In 2007, 142 million acres were planted in the United States alone.
- Monsanto uses extremely aggressive tactics on small farmers who are accused of using their seeds without permission, who voice serious concerns about the health risks of GMO's, and who refuse to participate in this business practice and model.

According to an article by Aurora Geib titled: "GMO Alert: Top 10 Genetically Modified Foods to Avoid Eating", you can buy the below products organically and without genetic modifications.

- Corn
- Soy
- Cotton
- Papaya
- Rice
- Tomatoes
- Rapeseed (Canola Oil)
- Dairy Products
- Potatoes
- Peas

There is no way to know what food has been genetically altered. The biotech companies have worked tirelessly and with great success to prevent any type of regulation making them accountable to the general public about which foods have been genetically altered. We are the guinea pigs in regard to the health risks associated with this type of farming and science. Our children are the first in this country's history to be barraged by ingredients in their packaged foods that have been genetically altered.

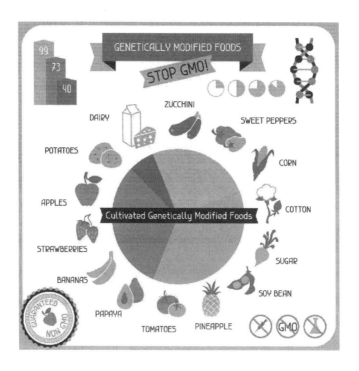

And we wonder why our children face so many medical, behavioral, and neurological issues today. It is possible before a fruit or vegetable gets to our plate for breakfast, lunch, or dinner it has been sprayed with a chemical pesticide, grown in soil that contains hazardous waste, and is now genetically altered. Wow!

Suggestions:
- Buy organic and locally grown produce (ask questions though)
- Grow your own garden
- Reduce the amount of foods you and your family consume that have high levels of pesticide residue
- Thoroughly wash produce
- Remove outer layer or leaf before eating
- Reduce or eliminate pesticides used on your lawn or in your garden

---

References

1. Grace Communications Foundation, Pesticides, Accessed on May 17, 2011, http://www.sustainabletable.org/issues/pesticieds/

2. Grace Communications Foundation, Pesticides, Accessed on May 8, 2014, http://www.sustainabletable.org/263/pesticides

3. Harmful Farm Chemicals, Accessed on May 7, 2011, http://www.ehow.com/list_6816618_harmful-farm-chemicals.html

4. Rodale Institute, "A Growing Concern: Hazardous Waste in Fertilizer", Accessed on May 20, 2011, http://newfarm.rodaleinstitute.org/depts/gleanings/0803/rutter.shtml.

5. United States Environmental protection Agency, "How many people work for the EPA?", Accessed on May 8, 2014, http://publicaccess.supportportal.com/link/portal/23002/23012/article/17588/how-many-people-work-for-the-EPA

6. United States Environmental Protection Agency, EPA's Budget and Spending, Accessed on May 8, 2014, http://www2.epa.gov/planandbudget/budget

7. United States Environmental Protection Agency, Wastes- Hazardous Waste, Accessed on May 20, 2011, http://www.epa.gov/waste/hazard/index.htm

8. Fair Measures, Inc., "Killing Fields? Toxic waste being spread as fertilizer", Accessed on May 20, 2011, http://www.fairmeasures.com/ask/enews/archive/summer97/new08.asp

9. Voice Of The Environment, "The Poisoning of America's Farmlands: From Toxic Waste to Fertilizer to Our Food Supply", Accessed on July, 25, 2011, http://www.voiceoftheenvironment.org/poisoning_farmlands/

10. Environmental Working Group, Toxic Wastes "Recycled" As Fertilizer Threatens U.S. Farms and Food Supply, Accessed on May 8, 2014, http://www.ewg.org/news-releases/1998/05/26/toxic-wastes-recycled-fertilizer-threatens-us-farms-and-food-supply

11. Environment California, Environmental Health reports, Accessed on May 20, 2011, http://www.environmentcalifornia.org/reports/environmental-health/environmental-health-reports/as-you-sow-toxic-waste-in-california-home-and-farm-fertilizer

12. United States Federal Drug Administration, Food, Accessed on May12, 2014, http://www.fda.gov/Food.FoodScienceResearch/Biotechnology/ucm346030.htm

13. HealthCastle.com, "Genetically Modified Foods: Hearing Both Sides of the Story", Accessed on June 13, 2011, http://www.healthcastle.com/genetically_modified_foods.shtml

14. Vanity Fair, "Monsanto's Harvest of Fear", Accessed on May 17, 2011, http://www.vanityfair.com/politics/features/2008/05/monsanto200805

15. ProQuest, "Genetically Modified Foods: Harmful or Helpful?", Accessed on May 12, 2014, http://www.csa.com/discoveryguides/gmfood/overview.php

16. Huffington Post, "Round-up Birth Defects: Regulators Knew World's Best-Selling Herbicide Causes Problems, New Report Finds", Accessed on June 7, 2011, http://www.huffingtonpost.com/2011/06/07/round-up-birth-defects-herbicides-regulators_n_872862.html

17. Non-GMO Project, What is GMO? Agricultural Crops that Have a Risk of Being GMO, Accessed on May 12, 2014, http://www.nongmoproject.org/learn-more/what-is-gmo/

18. Non-GMO Project, GMO Facts Frequently Asked Questions, Accessed on May 12, 2014, http://www.nongmoproject.org/learn-more/

19. Institute for Responsible Technology, Health Risks, Accessed on May 12, 2014, http://responsibletechnology.org/health-risks

20. Organic Consumers Association, "Spilling the Beans: Unintended GMO Health Risks", Accessed on May 12, 2014, http://www.organicconsumers.org/articles/article_11361.cfm

21. Organic Consumers Association, Monsanto's Government Ties, Accessed on May 12, 2014, http://www.organicconsumers.org/monsanto/news.cfm

22. Mindfully.org, "The Revolving Door, US Government Workers & University Researchers Go Biotech and Back Again. A Question of Ethics", Accessed on May 12, 2014, http://www.mindfully.org/GE/Revolving-Door.htm

23. Red Ice Creations, Monsanto's Government Ties, Accessed on May 12, 2014, http://www.redicecreations.com/specialreports/monsanto.html

24. Natural News, "GMO Alert: top 10 genetically modified foods to avoid eating", Accessed May 12, 2014, http://www.naturalnews.com/035734_gmos_foods_dangers.html

CHAPTER 11
The Chemicals That Make Our Food Look, Smell, and Taste Good

"We are living in a world today where lemonade is made from artificial flavors and furniture polish is made from real lemons."

—Alfred E. Newman

This chapter explores the specific ingredients found in our "everyday" packaged, processed, and frozen foods.

Chemical Preservatives/Food Dyes/ Artificial Ingredients

The preservation of food is not a new concept. For thousands of years people have come up with new ways and ideas on how to successfully preserve food for use at a later time. Salting meats, freezing, boiling, smoking, vacuum-packing, and dehydration have all been used to prevent food from spoiling. Included in some of these techniques is the use of sugar, vinegar, and alcohol. The processes and the ingredients mentioned above are considered natural preservatives. For the remainder of this section, I am emphasizing the synthetic and toxic chemicals added to our food today to preserve or enhance them.

Food additives such as artificial preservatives and food dyes are added to our food for several reasons. We are told this is done to prevent spoilage and improve color, texture, and taste. Preservatives can prevent the natural decomposition of fresh foods and mask the overgrowth of molds, fungus, and microorganisms in many food products. The key word is mask. Foods can stay on grocery store shelves for years due to the preservatives used to maintain their freshness and keep them from spoiling and going bad. More than 14,000 chemicals are now being added to our food supply including 3,000 food additives, preservatives, flavorings, and colorings. Preservatives increase the shelf life and appearance of foods that are fresh, frozen, and packaged. Some preservatives and artificial ingredients used in this process can be considered toxic or poisonous to our bodies. They are harmful to the body and can cause a number of health problems when consumed in large amounts and over a number of years. Some common food preservatives used in the United States have been banned in other countries due to the potential harm they can cause to humans. While there are limited studies on the effects of these chemicals on humans, laboratory animals have not been so lucky.

The chemically induced artificial preservatives, colorings, and ingredients used in our food today include:

Preservatives:

1. **BHA and BHT** (Butylated Hydroxyanisole and Butlylated Hydrotoluene): These are the two preservatives most often used in our food today. They are made from petroleum or coal tar.

Found in: pork products, potato chips, chewing gum, vegetable oils, snack foods, pies, processed meats, cake mixes, and cereals.

Also found in: embalming fluid and jet fuel.

Problem: These preservatives have caused cancer in rats. BHT is stored in human fat cells and may result in asthma, rhinitis, dermatitis, and tumors. BHA is thought to be a carcinogen to humans. They have both been found to alter brain chemistry in mice. The UK bans BHT from baby foods. BHA and BHT are banned completely in Japan and parts of the European Union.

2. Sodium Nitrates: Sodium nitrate is a naturally occurring salt and is used to preserve meat.

Found in: bacon, sausage, deli meats, hot dogs, bologna, corn beef, pepperoni, and smoked fish,

Also Found in: fertilizers to kill rodents and contaminated drinking water.

Problem: During the curing process, sodium nitrate and sodium nitrite are broken down into nitrosamines. Nitrosamines are carcinogenic. According to the Environmental Protection Agency, exposure to high levels of sodium nitrate has been linked to increased incidences of cancer in adults and may be related to brain tumors, leukemia, and nose and throat tumors in some children. Some infants develop "blue baby Syndrome" which is named for the blue color of their skin". A few studies have also reported an increased incidence of childhood diabetes, recurrent diarrhea, an increased risk of nervous system defects, respiratory tract infections, and possible increases of heart disease.

3. Caramel: This is a chemical color added to certain foods and beverages to enhance the color of a certain food. Caramel coloring is the single most used food coloring in the world. It is not a necessary ingredient and is used to make a product more appealing to our eyes.

Found in: bread, candy, brown colored food, frozen pizza, and colas.

Problem: Caramel coloring is the result of reacting sugar with ammonia and sulfites under high pressure and temperatures. The chemical reaction creates

2-methylimidazole and 4-methylimidazole. In government conducted studies they cause lung, liver, and thyroid cancer and leukemia in mice or rats. Caramel coloring has the potential to affect enzymes, RNA, and thyroid functioning. Chemicals that cause cancer in animals are considered to pose cancer threats to humans. In 2007, a federal government study concluded both of these cause cancer in mice. In 2011, the International Agency for Research on Cancer determined they are "possible" carcinogenic to humans. Consumer Reports conducted a study on popular soda brands and determined that the amount of caramel coloring in sodas carried varying levels of these carcinogens. For example, Sprite contained no significant levels of 4-Mel, Coke contained under 4 micrograms and Pepsi, diet Pepsi, and Pepsi One contained much higher levels. Malta and Goya contained the highest amount and far exceeded the amount deemed safe by this report. The California Office of Environmental Health Hazard Assessment used 29 micrograms per can as the cut-off point because that's the level they determined poses a one in one hundred thousand risk of cancer per individual who consume at least 29 micrograms daily for a lifetime.

4. Artificial flavors: This chemical ingredient is used to mimic a natural flavor found in a specific food. Companies are experimenting in laboratory settings with different chemicals and chemical compounds that eventually make their way into our food supply.

Found in: most packaged and processed foods.

Problem: They are linked to allergic reactions, eczema, hyperactivity, and asthma.

5. Artificial Sweeteners: Artificial sweeteners are highly processed and chemically derived zero calorie sweeteners found in diet foods and diet products to reduce calories per serving.

Types of artificial sweeteners include: Acesulfame-K, Aspartame (NutraSweet and equal), Saccharine, Sucralose, and sorbitol.

Found in: pharmaceutical products, supplements, toothpaste, diet drinks, diet foods, ice cream, gum, and yogurts.

Problem: These products can negatively impact metabolism and some have been linked to cancer, dizziness, hallucinations, and headaches.

6. Sodium Benzoate/Potassium Benzoate/Benzoic Acid: These preservatives preserve fats and prevent foods from becoming rancid.

Found in: pickles, flour, margarine, fruit purees and juices, beer, soft drinks, tea, coffee, and almost all fast food hamburgers.

Problem: Sodium benzoate can combine with vitamin C to form benzene, a highly carcinogenic compound. The risk of cancer to humans is low if that makes you feel any better. This group of chemical food preservatives has been banned in Russia because of its role in triggering allergies, asthma, and skin conditions. The FDA has urged (not mandated) companies not to use this additive. Most companies continue to use it today. This preservative may also cause brain damage.

7. Bromate (Potassium Bromate): This additive increases the volume of bread and produces a fine crumb.

Found in: foods that contain flour.

Problem: Most bromate breaks down into bromide which is OK. Bromate itself causes cancer in animals. Bromate has been banned virtually worldwide except for Japan and the United States. California requires a warning label on foods containing bromates. It can also cause nutrient deficiencies, diarrhea, and has been linked to kidney and nervous system disorders.

8. Sulfites: Sulfites are a class of chemicals that keep cut-up fruits and vegetables looking fresh, prevent dark spots on shrimp, and prevent bacterial growth and fermentation in wine.

Found in: fruit, dried fruit, jarred olives and peppers, corn syrup, cornstarch, wine vinegar, and wine.

Problem: Sulfites may cause headaches, joint pain, heart palpitations, allergies, and cancer.

9. Monosodium Glutamate (MSG): MSG is a chemically derived flavor enhancer and is made from the sodium salt of glutamic acid.

Found in: soups, dressings, chips, frozen entrees, broths, gravies, canned and frozen meats, fish, poultry, vegetables, ketchup, soy sauce, sausages, and snack foods.

Problem: While MSG is considered a safe chemical by the USDA, according to Russell Blaylock, author of a book entitled, *Excitotoxins: the Taste That Kills*, MSG is considered an excitotoxin which means this preservative excites the neurons in the brain. Blaylock states that excitotoxins may aggravate many neurological disorders such as Alzheimer's and Parkinson's disease. Side effects of MSG may include: seizures, allergies, rashes, asthma attacks, headaches, and brain tumors. It can also cause numbness, chest pains, drowsiness, and tingling. The food industry is hiding this ingredient in your food under the following names: hydrolyzed vegetable protein, hydrolyzed protein, sodium caseinate, calcium caseinate, bouillon, gelatin, malt extract and flavoring, broth, stock, seasoning, spices, and soy protein concentrate and isolate.

10. **Food dyes:** This is a liquid or powder added to a food or drink to change or enhance its color and appearance. Food dyes are what make candies and certain foods attractive and bright in color. There are several artificial dyes approved for use in food by the United States Food and Drug Administration (FDA). These include:

FD&C Blue No. 1
FD&C Blue No. 2
FD&C Green No. 3
FD&C Red No. 40
FD&C Red No. 3
FD&C Yellow No. 5
FD&C Yellow No. 6

There are two other artificial food colorings that have restricted use:
Orange B is a coloring allowed only in the casings of hot dogs and sausages.
Citrus Red Number 2 is allowed for coloring the skins of oranges.

There have been several artificial food dyes the FDA originally approved for use in foods that have been deemed unsafe for human consumption and are no longer used today. They include Red Number 2, 4, and 32; Orange Numbers 1 and 2; Yellow Numbers 1, 2, 3, and 4; and Violet Number 1.

The most extensive report on food dyes and their effect I found in my research is compiled by (CSPI) The Center for Science in the Public Interest titled, "Food Dyes – A Rainbow of Risk". If you would like to read this report in its entirety please go to www.cspinet.org/nw/pdf/food-dyes-rainbow-of-risk.pdf. This study states that almost all the toxicological studies on the specific dyes were commissioned, conducted, and analyzed by the chemical industry. The chemical industry is responsible for making the dyes and selling these food colorings to the multi-national food companies. The report's final conclusion is all of these food dyes need to be banned from human consumption and further independent testing be conducted. According to this report, the health problems associated with the seven current food dyes approved for use in the United States that are based on the experiments conducted with laboratory rats and mice include: an increase in kidney tumors, brain tumors, tumors of the urinary bladder, testicle tumors, adrenal tumors, and an increase in thyroid carcinogens. Other concerns related to our children's overall health include: a potential increase in hyperactivity, attention concerns, anxiety, migraines, increased risk of cancer, hypersensitivity, allergic reactions, and behavioral maladies.

These studies and their conclusions were conducted solely on one specific food dye at a time. Most of the processed foods we consume contain more than one food dye. There is limited research on the effects of these chemicals being combined together in the same product. The FDA should ban food dyes which serve no purpose other than a cosmetic one. Loopholes in the law make it difficult to ban this ingredient. CSPI also has an updated guide to food additives called Chemical Cuisine. This can be reviewed at www.nutritionaction.com/shop/chemical-cuisine-your-guide-to-food-additives/.

Europe is much further along than we are in the United States in regard to the fact that chemicals are negatively affecting our children who are consuming large quantities of them in their food each and every day. These countries have stricter laws regarding the chemicals that can be added to food. Below is a simple example of the difference a few ingredients can make in the quality of a product. One box is sold in the United States and the other one in Europe. It is the same product made by the same company, yet the ingredients are significantly different.

Kellogg's Nutri-Grain bars are made with natural colorings in Britain but contain food dyes in the United States. It is the same product by the same company.

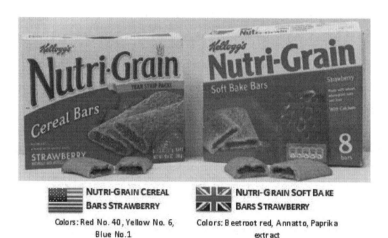

	NUTRI-GRAIN CEREAL BARS STRAWBERRY		NUTRI-GRAIN SOFT BAKE BARS STRAWBERRY
	Colors: Red No. 40, Yellow No. 6, Blue No.1		Colors: Beetroot red, Annatto, Paprika extract

Photo Credit: CSPI

It seems overwhelming with the number of issues that are a cause for concern in our food supply. However, things are changing for the better. Yes, there are significant health concerns regarding the way in which food companies are producing food and the chemicals they are adding to the products we and our children consume on a daily basis. The list of concerns is long, extensive, and backed up by scientific research.

Currently, our food supply is unhealthy and contributing to disease on a level never before seen. Who is to blame? Do we place blame on the chemical companies, the food companies, the agricultural companies, the pharmaceutical companies or the government? How about all of them and include us as a responsible party for letting this happen. Money rules this country and the more we make the better, even if it causes harm to others. Our lives are dictated and controlled by the amount of money we make and little attention is given to the fact that we have created an environment that is toxic to EVERYONE! However, the good news is people are beginning to wake up on a massive scale. I know these companies probably follow the laws as authorized by the United States government. It is a standard that is dangerous to us all. We are the guinea pigs. Our children are the guinea pigs. We are losing! Our bodies cannot tolerate this systemic slow poisoning. Our bodies were not designed to process the types of foods that have become commonplace. We can, however, help our bodies keep a better balance.

There are companies and products available that reduce, significantly reduce, or eliminate most of the concerns brought to your attention in the last few chapters and outside of this book. We no longer need to follow what is "normal" and can decide on purchasing food products that make sense and do not cause us harm. The food industry and what they are producing is very slowly changing. One only has to look at the amount of organic foods now sold in most grocery stores all across this country. I believe we owe it to our children to educate and teach them about all of these dangers. It is critical this craziness stops. To me it is craziness on an absurd and monumental level. These companies are knowingly poisoning the American population as a whole. Why? Why is the government allowing this to happen? Who is working for us and do we individually and collectively have the guts, determination, and fortitude to say no more? Can we accept change in our lives and begin to look at things from a different perspective? Can we stand up and say that enough is enough? If these corporations hurt one of us, they hurt all of us. There is no division here. Whew. I have said my peace.

Now that we are aware of some of the dangers a few of the chemicals mentioned in this book have on our bodies, imagine the magnitude of the problem if we discussed the thousands of chemicals used to supposedly "enhance" our food and lives. The next few chapters will help you begin to make some changes. Becoming aware is the first step. Let's see how you can transform your kitchen and mindset in a way that reduces this stuff.

Reference

1. BRIGHT HUB, "Harmful Effects of Food Preservatives", Accessed on June 16, 2011, http://www.brighthub.com/health/alternative-medicine/articles/42704.aspx

2. Nutritious You, Harmful Effects of Food Preservatives, Accessed on May 12, 2014, http://raw.marinasommers.com/2009/12/food-preservatives.html

3. Newsmax health, "10 things Americans Eat That Are Banned in Other Countries", Accessed on May 13, 2014, htto://www.newsmaxhealth.com/headline/banned-food-preservatives-carcinogenic/2014/04/22/Id/566896/

4. Food Identity Theft, "A pair of preservatives you need to be aware of", Accessed on May 14, 2014, http://foodidentitytheft.com/a-pair-of-preservatives-you-need-to-be-aware-of/-the-top-ten-additives-to-avoid-countdown-continues/

5. Livestrong.com, 10 Worst Food Additives, Accessed on May 1, 2014, http://www.livestrong.com/article/470375-10-worst-food-additives/

6. Livestrong.com, The Most Common Food Preservative, Accessed on May 13, 2014, http://www.livestrong.com/article/288335-the-most-common-food-preservatives/

7. Mercola.com, U.S. Foods Chockfull of Ingredients Banned in Other Countries, Accessed on May 13, 2014, http://articles.mercola.com/sites/articles/archive/2013/02/27/us-food-products.aspx

8. Center For Science In The Public Interest, Food Dyes: A Rainbow of Risks, Accessed on June 16, 2014, http://www.cspinet.org/new/pdf/food-dyes-rainbow-of-risks.pdf

9. Sweet poison, Food Additives to Avoid, Accessed on June 16, 2011, http://www.sweetpoison.com/food-additives-to-avoid.html

10. Mayo Clinic, Does the Sodium nitrate in processed meats increase my risk of heart disease>, Accessed on May 14, 2014, http://www.mayoclinic.org/healthy-living/nutrition-and-healthy-eating/expert-answers/sodium-nitrate/faq-20057848

11. Environmental Protection Agency, Nitrates and Nitrites, Accessed on February 23, 2013, http://www.epa.gov/teach/chem_summ/Nitrates_summary.pdf

12. Center For Science In The Public Interest, FDA Urged to Prohibit Carcinogenic "caramel Coloring", http://www.cspinet.org/new/201102161.html

13. The Huffington Post, Caramel Coloring in Soda: What You Should Know About This Innocent-Sounding Ingredient, Accessed on May 14, 2014, http://www.huffingtonpost.com/michael-f-jacobson/caramel-coloring-in-soda_b_823639.html

14. Consumer Reports, Caramel Color: The health risk that may be in your soda, Accessed on May 14, 2014, http://www.consumerreports.org/cro/news/2014/01/caramel-color-the-health-risk-that-may-be-in-your-soda/index.htm

15. Food Safety News, "Consumer Reports Study Prompts FDA to Reexamine Caramel Coloring", Accessed on May 14, 2014, http://www.foodsafetynews.com/2014/01/fda-to-reexamine-caramel-coloring-in-sodas-due-to-impurity/#.U3OIiMu9KSM

16. U, S Food And Drug Administration, Summary of Color Additives for Use in the UNITED States in Food, Drugs, Cosmetics, and Medical Devices, Accessed on May 14, 2014, http://www.fda.gov/forindustry/coloradditives/coloradditiveinventories/ucm115641.htm

17. Science News, Artificial Food Coloring Dangers, Accessed on May 13, 2014, http://science-news.org/artificial -food-coloring/artificial-food-coloring-dangers/

18. Forbes, "Living in Color: The Potential Dangers of Artificial Dyes", Accessed on May 13, 2014, http://www.forbes.com/sites/rachelhennessey/2012/08/27/living-in-color-the-potential-dangers-of-artificial-dyes/

19. Mercola.com, Are You or Your Family Eating Toxic Food Dyes, Accessed on May 13, 2014, http://articles.mercola.com/sites/articles/archive/2011/02/24/are-you-or-your-family-eating-toxic-food-dyes.aspx

20. Absolute Astronomy, Food Coloring, Accessed on June 22, 2011, http://www.absoluteastronomy.com/topics/Food_coloring

21. Center For Science In The Public Interest, Food Dyes, Accessed on August 4, 2011, http://www.cspinet.org/fooddyes/

22. Web MD, the Truth about 7 Common Food Additives, Accessed on June 22, 2011. http://wwww.webmd.com/diet/features/the-truth-about-seven-common-food-additives

23. Science News, Artificial Food Coloring Dangers, Accessed on October 20, 2010, http://science-news.org/artifical-food-coloring/artificial-food-coloring-dangers/f

Section 3
What Can I Do?

"If nothing ever changed, there'd be no butterflies."

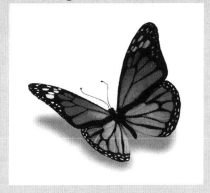

~Author Unknown

I have two schools of thought for parents as they continue learning more about these very important topics. First, if you have a child or children suffering from autism, asthma, allergies (food and environmental), behavioral problems, diabetes, ADD/ADHD, emotional problems, obesity, learning disabilities, digestive disorders, constant ear infections, colds and flu-like symptoms, mental health issues, or other explained and unexplained daily physical symptoms, let me tell you right here and now, welcome to the club. No parent wants or wishes to be a part of this club. The important thing to understand is that you are not alone. More and more of us are frustrated with not getting answers from the medical community. Keep researching, reading, and asking questions. I am assuming you have made it to this point because you just don't know what else to do and began researching other options. This journey may have been long, dark, daunting, and overwhelming, but here you stand. Each of our journeys, our children's journeys, and our bodily health may be different. However, we are all coming to the same conclusions. We are all gaining a basic understanding of how our bodies work and what we need to do to help our child control or eliminate his or her symptoms. One of these ways is to look at foods as a way to reduce or eliminate symptoms. Be proud of the steps you have taken to help your child and continue on toward finding the answers for the questions you want answered.

I will not be providing the exact treatment plan that I followed for my son because all of our children are different in terms of symptoms and needs. I am suggesting to you though that some childhood illnesses and diseases have the potential to have two things in common. The two common concerns are Candida (chronic yeast infection) and toxic and chemical sensitivity and overload. Your child would benefit greatly from an alternative approach to treating disease (some of these alternative approaches might include acupuncture, nutrition counseling, Chinese medicine, aromatherapy, herbal medicine, counseling, massage, holistic or functional medicine, and homeopathy or naturopathic medicine). How about an integrated approach to the medical treatment of your child by using modern medicine and alternative treatment plans in combination for optimal health? To learn more about alternative medicine options go to http://altmedworld.net/alternative.htm. Your child will benefit greatly from nutritional support and education. It truly works! I am suggesting you continue searching for the right practitioner to help you in this journey. They are out there waiting to help you transform your child's life. I am sure, just like me, that you have absolutely nothing to lose by taking a different approach to your child's symptoms. You are on the right track! The resource section of this book will identify practitioners in your area to assist you.

The other school of thought is for parents who have no immediate or chronic health concerns regarding their child or children. You may have found this book by accident or it was given to you by a friend. Either way, it is my hope that you will offer compassion and love to your family and friends that have children who are suffering with some of the diseases and symptoms described throughout this book. It can be a very lonely and heartbreaking journey for parents. I also hope that you will look at the issues laid out in this book as an opportunity to remain or become mindful of your own family's health. You are blessed and have the opportunity to be proactive in regard to these issues. There is no physical disease or on-going symptom(s) that require immediate attention. You can take a calculated and systematic approach to this process of change.

This section of the book will offer suggestions and resources for your own home. I suggest marking all of the ideas or resources that resonate with you today. Everything you read in the remainder of this book may not resonate with you on a personal level. If it does great, but if not, that is OK as well.

My suggestions to help get you started include:

1. Take an hour and walk around your house. Look in your cabinets, refrigerator, freezer, bathroom closets, and under your sinks. Read the labels. What do you want to change or eliminate? What can you change or eliminate?

2. Are you concerned with the consumption of the tap water in your home?

3. Are you concerned with the air quality in your home?

4. Write a food journal. For one week write down everything that you or your child eats. You will begin to see a pattern emerge. You will be able to get a better sense of what your child's nutritional intake looks like on a day-to-day basis.

5. If appropriate, begin speaking to your spouse or significant other about the changes you want to make and why. They have to be willing to work with you

or it will become a more difficult goal or process for you to achieve. However, it can be done.

6. Sit down with your child once you have a plan of action and discuss your new ideas with him or her.

7. Think about the physical and emotional concerns you have in regard to your children. Do you see a pattern of behavior or a pattern of unhealthy eating? Does your child suffer from chronic symptoms, a disease, or a neurological disorder? What behaviors do you see on a day-to-day basis?

8. How often is your child taking a medication or an antibiotic?

9. Do you want to make your environment healthier for your family?

10. Begin researching topics that you can relate to or that you are concerned about.

CHAPTER 12
One Step of Change at a Time

*"Let food be thy medicine, thy medicine
shall be thy food."*
—HIPPOCRATES

How can you eliminate the junk food and unnecessary chemicals from your child's diet and environment? Specifically, what can you add or replace something with that is a healthier option? I have included a few helpful hints as you begin to navigate your way around the maze of major grocery store chains, national food companies, and the vast array of options that are awaiting you.

I am going to jump right in, but please remember that if you have decided to make some changes, this is a process. I did not implement all of these changes overnight. It is still a work in progress for me. Your changes do not have to be my changes. I learn something new all the time about the foods we eat. My food and environmental choices have evolved slowly. It might make sense to create a sense of accomplishment by first looking at and changing the cleaning supplies and beauty products that you use today. Once you are comfortable with those changes, you can then begin to replace foods.

How to get started:

Take advantage of the pages in the beginning of this book that asks for your written responses. Complete the questionnaires to give you the feedback you need to get started. List the changes you are looking to make, if any. Identify in your daily environment the foods, chemicals, and toxins you want to eliminate for your family. I have included some helpful hints below that I have learned over the last five years to help you in this process. These suggestions can help you achieve your desires as you navigate your way around the grocery store.

• Shop in the outer perimeter of the store:

The first thing I noticed about my shopping habit that changed dramatically over time is that I found myself no longer shopping in the aisles, but in the perimeter or outer part of the grocery store. The perimeter of the store is where you will find the healthier and perishable foods.

However, some stores combine conventional products and organic products together in the same shelf space in the middle aisles of the store. If this is the case, pick an item that you are going to purchase, take a minute, and look around for its healthier or organic version.

• Shop in the "organic" section of the store:

Most grocery stores now have an aisle or two of organic foods. Grocery stores only carry food items that consumers purchase. It is a good sign stores and companies are giving more shelf space to healthier foods. Consumers are demanding it! Stores are developing their own organic brand to compete in the organic marketplace.

Almost every food corporation and grocery store chain today realizes that the organic food industry is worth billions of dollars a year in sales. It is a "new" market in which to make a lot of money. In 2001, the sales of organic foods and beverages exceeded $9 billion dollars. In 2009, the sales of organic foods topped $24 billion dollars. Another study in 2009 suggests that organic product sales reached $26.6 billion dollars. The U.S. organic industry grew by 9.5 percent in 2011 to reach $31.5 billion in sales. Of this, the organic food and beverage sector accounted for $29.22 billion and the non-organic food sector reached $2.2 billion dollars. According to the Nutrition Business Journal, organic sales in the United States grew from approximately $11 billion in 2004 to an estimated $27 billion in 2012. The specific number will always be changing and will depend on your source. The common factor with these current numbers is that this sector of food products is growing and quickly. The "organic" food sector is increasing each and every year.

Some companies produce organic foods because they value the principle of health for individuals and the environment. On the other hand, some of the huge food companies are now producing organic products because of the shift in consumer demand and because of the fact that big money and profit is involved. It is your choice to determine which companies you would like to give your hard earned money to.

I do not want to imply that the word "organic" suggests that it is 100 percent perfect. It is not. It is a better option than most of the other options vying for your attention and money.

The expansion of the organic industry has greatly reduced the cost of products, but read the labels. Just because something says it is "natural" doesn't necessarily mean it is good for us. Everybody now wants to get a piece of the profit from healthier foods, not because they have made a moral decision to make quality food, but because the bottom dollar says it is a good strategy.

Below are some examples of stores and their own brand of organic food.

Wegmans – Wegmans Organic
Giant/Stop & Shop – Nature's Promise
Target – Archer Farm
Kroger – Private Selections
Safeway – Wild Harvest
Publix – Green Wise
Whole Foods – 365
Winn Dixie – Organics & Naturals

I recently spent an hour or so in both a local Target and Wal-Mart store to determine and analyze the organic food choices in an effort to compare selections of organic foods for you. I typically do not purchase food from these companies, but know everyone has these stores in their community. I chose not to include Wal-Mart in the lists I provide for you because I found their selection of organic food to be limited and their botanical cleaning supplies to be minimal. Target, on the other hand, had a much wider selection of food items and beauty and cleaning supplies. My suggestion would be to use your grocery store and Target when making the necessary changes. If you live next to a Whole Foods or health food store that is an added bonus.

- Stop or reduce buying all of the processed and packaged foods that are specifically marketed to children.
  The colors of the food and its packaging are geared to capture our attention and they do. The problem is that while corporations have spent millions of dollars to advertise their products to our children, the products are unhealthy and contain toxic chemicals. The ironic thing is now these very same companies are producing organic foods. You can now buy a cookie from the same company that is highly processed or a cookie that is organic with fewer ingredients. They are catering to two very different consumers.

- Do not become overwhelmed.
  Take it slow and you will succeed. (I had absolutely no idea what I was doing when I began this transformation). Making any change is a step in the right direction.

- Reduce the number of ingredients found in a specific product and see if you can afford to buy organic.
  Start reading food labels. The fewer ingredients listed the better. I would stay away from or reduce products that contain high fructose corn syrup, soy, corn, and gluten. Eliminating these ingredients will greatly reduce all processed foods.

- Look for meat that is organic or at the very least grass-fed.
  This is more expensive. I have cut back on the serving size. Meat should only be a small portion of your meal anyway. Maybe even choose to have one or two days without serving meat.

- Start your own garden.

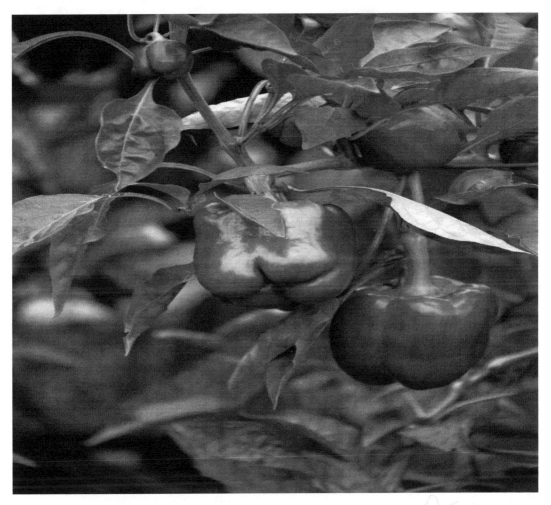

The kids love this idea and it makes them active participants in the changes you are trying to make. Start a small garden. As you become more comfortable and successful, increase the size of it.

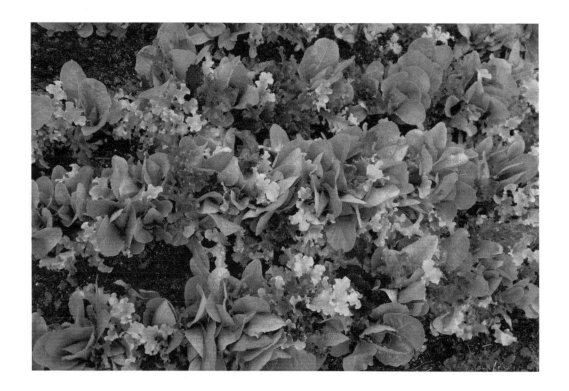

- Look at the possibility of farmers' markets in your area.

  You can go to www.localharvest.org to find a market close to your house. This website will pull up all of the farmers' markets in your area. Be sure to ask about the quality of the product before buying. Some products will be organic and others have been sprayed with pesticides and chemicals. The advantage of a farmers' market is that you are helping local farmers and your community. The food is fresh. It has not had to travel a far distance.

- Begin to eliminate artificial colors from your foods.

  Most conventional, kid friendly foods are loaded with food-dyes. Go for food that is more neutral in color except for fruits and vegetables.

    Some examples that I have used with my own children are:

    If they choose to get an ice cream cone, I try and eliminate the sprinkles (Can you serve them a dairy free frozen treat such as ice cream or chocolate pops made with coconut or almond milk?).

If they want potato chips in their lunch, I buy organic or plain. I have eliminated all of the ingredients that make up the flavored chips. Maybe now or in the future you can introduce sweet potato chips, veggie chips, gluten-free chips, bean chips, fresh kale chips, or make your own sprouted grain tortilla chips using sprouted grain tortillas.

If they want candy, I steer them toward something else like a healthier cookie. I have eliminated a lot of the artificial colors and reduced the amount of sugar. Is it possible to provide a mini-meal, nuts, hummus, raw veggies, a bowl of soup, a salad, etc.?

- Reduce the amount of sugar your child is consuming on a daily basis.
  It might be beneficial to complete a one week food journal of your child's current food habits. Write down the food consumed and be sure to include drinks. This will give you a better indication of how much sugar your child is actually consuming. The journal will assist you in identifying the areas for needed change. You will be amazed at how much sugar your child is actually consuming. I was!

- Reduce or eliminate milk and dairy products you serve your child on a daily basis. You can substitute milk for almond or coconut milk. At the very least, you can substitute it in your baking. They will never taste the difference.

- If you do not want to eliminate dairy, buy dairy products labeled organic. This includes yogurt and cheeses. How about serving your children organic milk and maybe just cut down on the amount given?

- Introduce more fish into your diet
  I know there is a concern about the toxicity of fish nowadays. I would suggest not buying farm raised fish and to ask about the quality of the fish such as whether there are chemicals used to add color to the fish and what part of the world it comes from? An informative website to explore this issue is www.seafoodwatch.org.

Since most fish carry varying levels of mercury, I would limit your fish intake to 1-3 servings a week. Fish with the lowest levels of mercury include catfish, haddock, halibut, salmon, snapper and trout. Shellfish (clams, oysters, shrimp, crab, scallops and lobster) can be full of toxins because they are scavengers or bottom dwellers and often feed off of the waste of other fish and sources of sewage.

- Drink plenty of good quality water.

Decrease or eliminate all sugar drinks. Children tend not to drink enough water in a given day and by eliminating alternatives you increase the possibility of adequate water consumption. Find a good, clean source. I am going out on a limb to say that tap water is not the best option for quality water. Most municipalities add chemicals such as fluoride and chlorine to the water supply. Maybe make a soda or juice a treat every once in a while?

If your children are young this transformation will be less challenging for you. Your transformation will be easier because your children won't know any differently. You can set the stage for proper nutrition and educate your children from a young age. I would suggest holding a family meeting to discuss your new ideas on food with your children, if they are age appropriate. Develop a plan together. I would be open about the concerns you have with the foods they are eating and develop strategies. It is important to include your children in this process and become educated together. Decide as a family what is going to be eliminated from the grocery list and why. Take them with you to the store and have them read labels.

Please do not be mistaken. My children continue to struggle with these changes and it has been years now. Why would a teenager eat hummus and veggies when the societal norm is to eat candy bars, ice cream, chips, McDonald's, soda, and SUGAR? I just continue to talk with them (ignore the complaints as best as I can) and hope that at some point in their lives they are able to make the connection between foods that provide nutrients and vitality and foods that cause disease. It is a constant struggle for me with a sixteen year old, a fourteen year old, and a thirteen year old in the house. They prefer to eat this stuff. However, if

I don't buy it, they can't eat it at home. They are getting to the ages where I have less and less control. They are becoming independent individuals who have to make their own choices. I can guide and educate them though.

- Let your family and friends know the changes you are making. It will be helpful if they are on your side. Plus, you will be educating them at the same time. The more people begin to make change, the easier it will become for all of us.

- Let your child's school know as well.
  When my children were younger I sent them to school with alternative candy and food choices for birthday treats and parties. The more people talk about these issues, the more control we will have as parents. Is it possible for a student to bring a healthy snack for a birthday party instead of cupcakes, donuts, or other junk food items? I know, what's the big deal? I agree that it is OK to let our children enjoy treats on occasion. When you throw in all of the birthday treats for every child and include all of the parties such as Valentine's Day, Halloween, Thanksgiving, Christmas, St. Patrick's Day, and Easter it becomes excessive. Now add on all of the parties, celebrations, and holidays outside of school. Their bodies have to work extremely hard to balance the sugar, gluten, and chemicals they are ingesting. I am merely asking is it possible to begin to eliminate the highly processed foods our kids are eating on a daily basis.

- Reduce or eliminate the purchasing of school lunches and fast food.

- Think about adding nutritional value to your children's daily diet through vitamins and supplements.
  Let's face it, kids are picky eaters. I have one who will eat almost no vegetables and others who will eat minimal veggies. Vegetables provide an array of minerals and nutrients to their growing bodies. There are supplements to help if they are picky eaters. This approach should utilize a skilled practitioner to assist you.

- Increase the amounts of fruits and veggies (Buy organic when possible and refer back to pages 161-162 that list the fruits and vegetable most contaminated by pesticides.).

- Increase the amount of seeds and nuts your children are eating. They are high in protein, fiber, and good fat.

- I have found that buying in bulk once a month and going to the grocery store once a week, instead of several times, helps to reduce my grocery bills. I do make a second trip during the week to replenish the fruits and vegetables.

- Buying organic will be more expensive. You can refer to the websites in the next section of this book for online coupons. When you begin to reduce or eliminate some of the processed foods, sodas, and sugars from your grocery list, you can transfer that money to a few healthier items.

- You will probably notice that it takes a little bit longer to complete your grocery shopping in the beginning. That is OK. You will then notice it takes only a few minutes to find everything on your list. I would suggest that for the first few months you do the grocery shopping by yourself. This will give you a chance to get acclimated to where your family's new products are in the store. Once you are comfortable, invite your child to participate.

- Begin to understand that our bodies need certain foods in order to maintain proper and expanded nutritional balance. This includes the proper balance of acid vs. alkalinity in the blood (pH balance).

References

1. United States Department of Agriculture, Consumer demand drives growth in the organic sector, Accessed on May 14, 2014, http://www.ers.usda.gov/data-products/chart-gallery/detail.aspx?chartId=35003&.U3PrZcu9KSM

2. Organic trade Organization, 2010 Press Releases, U.S. Organic Product sales reached $26.6 billion in 2009, Accessed on June 9, 2011, http://www.organic newsroom.com/2010/04/us_organic_product_sales_reach_1.html

3. The Packer, "Organic fresh produce sales rise by 13% in 2012", Accessed on May 14, 2014, http://www.thepacker.com/fruit-vegetable-news/22580921.html

4. Organic Trade Organization, 2012 Press Release, "Consumer-driven U.S. organic market surpasses $31 billion in 2011, Accessed on May 14, 2014, http://www.organicnewsroom.com/2012/04/us_consumersdriven_organic_mark.html

CHAPTER 13
Organic Foods

"Chronic disease is a foodborne illness. We ate our way into this mess, and we must eat our way out."
—MARK HYMAN

It is important to understand what the term "organic" means in regard to food and your weekly trip to the grocery store. For an extensive (and overwhelming) evaluation of the term "organic," go to www.usda.gov for further research. I am trying to only highlight what I think is important as you begin to navigate your way through the food industry and the continuous black hole of information.

In 1990, Congress passed the Organic Foods Protection Act. This act requires the USDA to develop national standards for organically produced products. As consumers, we can simply look for the labels highlighted below to identify products that are organic. These labels can usually be found on the packaging and is most often displayed on the front of a package or box where it is most visible. This label can be found on raw, fresh, frozen, packaged, and processed products.

An organic product is one that has been produced without antibiotics, hormones, chemical pesticides, irradiation, bioengineering techniques (GMO's), synthetic or artificial ingredients (chemicals), and chemical fertilizers.

Both commercial farming and organic farming use pesticides in the management of their crops. The difference is that commercial farming uses synthetic chemicals and organic farming uses natural resources. Both conventional agriculture and organic agriculture have their problems. For example, rotenone is an organic pesticide that was used for years. It was banned in 2005 due to the potential health concerns, as it was linked to Parkinson Disease like symptoms in rats. Organic farming is not a panacea or cure for conventional farming. It makes up only a small amount of the food produced in this country. It is also land and labor intensive and costs more money to consumers. However, I firmly believe that organic is a better choice.

The USDA now uses private and state agencies to inspect and certify food companies that make and market organic foods. Organic foods must meet the same safety requirements as conventional foods. I am not sure if this makes me feel comfortable that the people who are in charge of monitoring conventional foods are also in charge of monitoring organic foods. I just hope they are doing their jobs effectively and thoroughly.

What is the difference between conventional farming and organic farming?

Conventional Farming	**Food Organic Farming/Food**
Apply chemical fertilizers (including hazardous waste) to promote plant growth.	Apply natural fertilizers such as manure or compost to feed soil and plants. Organic farmers are allowed to use chemicals that are derived from nature, meaning they are not man-made but already found in nature. These include sulfur (mineral), copper, sabadilla (comes from the seed of a lily), nicotine sulfate (a chemical derived from tobacco), bat poop, and alfalfa meal.

Erodes soil and potentially damages or poisons bodies of water. Crops are typically grown in same soil year after year.	Reduces pollution associated with farming and also conserves water and soil. Organic farmers seek to preserve biodiversity and local ecosystems. Crop rotation and mixed planting are better for soil and environment.
Uses Chemical herbicides, pesticides, and insecticides.	Uses crop rotation, hand-weeding, or mulch to manage weeds. Uses beneficial insects and birds, mating disruptions, or traps to reduce pests and disease.
Gives animals antibiotics, growth hormones, and medications to prevent disease. Livestock today is raised on factory farms.	Gives animals organic feed, a balanced diet, and cleaner housing. Livestock was given no antibiotics, growth hormones, or medications. Under the organic standards, these animals are supposed to be treated in a more humane way.
Uses irradiation.	Does not use irradiation.
Food is less nutritious.	Studies have demonstrated higher amounts of nutrients in some varieties of organic foods. Organic foods do not contain artificial colors, chemical preservatives, and are not genetically modified.

Four types of visual labeling to help you identify organic foods while shopping: These labels can be found on fresh, frozen and packaged foods.

1.

 100% Organic

(This label tells you that everything in this product is organic. There is nothing in it that is synthetic or man-made.)

2.

(This label is the label I notice the most in stores. Products with this label are certified as 95 percent organic.)

3.

Made with Organic Ingredients

(This statement can only be used on items that contain at least 70 percent organic ingredients. This certification means that although the majority of ingredients used in this product are organic, there may also be a high concentration of conventionally produced ingredients. There is no food label for this classification.)

4.

Less Than 75% Organic Ingredients

(This statement refers to the amount of organic ingredients in ingredient list only. There is no label for this classification.)

Again, the organic food industry is becoming big business for the food industry and the multi-national companies that produce our food. For example: Campbell's Soup now owns Wolfgang Puck's organic soups; M&M Mars owns Seeds of Change; General Mills owns Lara Bar, Food Should taste Good, Cascadian Farms, and Muir Glen; Smucker's owns Santa Cruz Organics and R.W Knudsen; Kraft owns Back To Nature; Dean owns Horizon; ConAgra owns Alexia foods; Kellogg's owns Bear Naked, Kashi, and Morningstar; and The Dannon Company owns Stonyfield Farm. The big companies have bought the smaller, more independent farmers and organic food producers.

You can also find labels and advertisements on food packaging that state gluten-free, egg free, dairy free, nut free, shellfish free, soy free, and non-GMO. The amount of labels touting the healthy benefits of the foods we consume is growing. It is a maze in and of itself. The "all natural" label can be misleading. It is a meaningless label in my mind. The FDA does not define this term and leaves it up to the companies to determine if they will use this label. For example, high fructose corn syrup comes from corn which is a natural product but it has been heavily processed, possibly genetically modified, and sprayed with pesticides. Another product may be natural but contains added salt and preservatives. When choosing breads look for whole grain or 100%whole wheat and not breads that state multigrain or made with whole grain (Can you decrease the amount of gluten in your diet?). When a meat label says "free range" please understand this defined term by the U.S. Department of Agriculture does not account for the amount, duration, and quality of outdoor access. Another misleading label I am seeing more and more is the actual serving size information on the packaging. The serving size can be a tiny or unrealistic amount. This is done to make the product appear healthier than it is.

Basically, companies are coming up with tricky marketing and advertising slogans that are not necessarily accurate and in your best interest. These companies spend millions and millions of dollars every year trying to "out trick" the consumer. Why? Why it is such a secret to know what is in the food we eat? They must be hiding something?

References

1. USDA-FDA Organic Foods, Organic Foods, Accessed on June 9, 2011, http://usda-fda.gov/Organic-nutrition.htm

2. LoveToKnow, "What Does Organic Mean", Accessed on may22, 2011, http://organic.lovetoknow.com/What_Does_Organic_Mean

3. Center for American Progress, its Easy Being Green: Organic vs. Conventional foods – The Gloves Come Off, Accessed on June 9, 2011. http://www.americanprogress.org/issues/green/news/2008/09/10/4933/its-easy-being-green-vs-conventional-foods-the-gloves-come-off/

4. United States Department of Agriculture, National Organic Program, Accessed on June 9, 2011, http://www.ams.usda.gov/AMSv1.0/ams.fetchTemplateData.do?template=TemplateA&navID=NationalOrganicProgram&leftNav=NationalOrganicProgram&page=NOPUnderstandingOrganicLabeling&description=Understanding%20Organic%20Labeling&acct=nopgeninfo

5. Cyber-Help for Organic Farmers, Who Owns What in the Organic food industry, Accessed on July 26, 2011, http://www.certifiedorganic.bc.ca/rcbtoa/services/corporate-ownership.html

6. Mercola.com. "What Giant Corporation Owns Your Favorite Organic food label, accessed on June 9, 2011, http://articles.mercola.com/sites/articles/archive/2008/04/01/which-giant-corporation-owns-your-favorite-organic-food-brand.aspx

CHAPTER 14
Out with the Old and In with the New

"We almost always have choice, and the better the choice, the more we will be in control."
—WILLIAM GLASSER

I have compiled the top twelve things or ideas to consider changing concerning toxins and chemicals in our food and environment. Some of these have been previously mentioned, but bear repeating. These suggestions might be the easiest things to consider changing and will greatly impact your family and your daily environment.

1. Water: Drink a lot of it and make sure it is clean. The number of filtering systems on the market today is high. You have to do your homework here. A product to consider is called Zero (www.zerowater.com). It looks similar to a Brita water pitcher and comes as both a water bottle and pitcher. It

has a five stage filtration system that reduces contaminants found in typical water. It is a relatively inexpensive water filtering system. Another product is a Dynamically Enhanced Natural Action Water Structuring Unit (www. naturalactiontechnologies.com). You can also research distilled water, reverse osmosis, and a commercially sold filtering system for your home and family.

2. Develop a better understanding of your digestive system. Educate yourself!

3. Cleaning and Beauty Supplies: Swap out chemically laden products with more organic or natural products. You can do this all at once or as you run out of a certain product.

4. Listen to your body—it does not lie! It is sending you messages all the time.

5. Buy organic when you can, as I believe it is a better choice all around.

6. Avoid foods that have been genetically modified. Until we are informed about what the health consequences are to our overall health, we should not be the guinea pigs.

7. Meats: Consider organic and grass-fed. Decrease or eliminate the amount of red meat in daily diet, pick lean cuts of meat, and increase your consumption of fish on occasion.

8. Decrease fast food, packaged, and processed foods.

9. Contact a nutritionist or homeopathic practitioner if you need assistance with your health.

10. Decrease products containing dairy, high fructose corn syrup, sugar, soy, and gluten.

11. Increase foods that are raw (fruits, vegetables, seeds, and nuts), nutrient-rich, and less chemically produced.

12. Eat veggies, veggies, and more veggies.

The list that begins for you on page 216 contains new products to consider when you shop. Your grocery store may carry its own organic brand not provided on the list below. The idea is to reduce or eliminate the chemicals from your food supply. The only way to do this is by changing your grocery spending habits and buying organic as much as possible. It is also important to consider simplifying your food intake. Think back a generation or two ago in your own family. The choices were more limited and there is something to be said for living off the land. God has provided all that has ever been needed to survive and thrive. If you cannot afford to buy all organic products, simply reduce the number of ingredients found in your packaged foods by reading labels.

The list of foods below does not take into account any specific dietary needs. Due to illnesses or symptoms, some people may have restrictive diets that limit or eliminate certain foods or ingredients from his or her diet. Certain digestive illnesses require a food rotation diet. Some people choose to be vegan (does not eat or wear anything of animal origin), vegetarian (eats no meat, but will eat eggs and dairy) or pescatarian (abstain from eating all meat, but will eat fish). The list below is geared more toward the "average" consumer who is willing and wanting to make some changes. I am not marginalizing anyone when I refer to the "average American consumer." I am merely trying to reach a specific audience with the changes in food selection that are described below. I have also included websites for your convenience. You can order foods and snacks directly from many companies online and in bulk.

I have eliminated or significantly reduced the following foods, ingredients, and chemicals from my home by reading labels, reducing processed and packaged foods, and buying organic.

Dairy

Corn and its' many derivatives, including HFCS

Sugar

Gluten

Artificial flavors and colors

Preservatives

Soy

Nitrates/nitrites/bromate/sulfites/MSG

Hormones (rBGH)

Antibiotic/steroid/fertilizer/pesticide residue

Chemicals found in cleaning supplies, water, and beauty supplies

GMO foods

BPA, BHA, BHT, and other synthetic chemicals

The items below are merely suggestions and examples of how you can replace processed food with a product that is a little bit healthier. I no longer purchase some of these specific foods items, but I wanted to give you as many options as I could find. I did not list all of the brands because this sector of the food business is growing at an exceptionally high rate of speed. New products are coming out all the time. You have to be careful and read labels in the beginning until you find exactly what you are looking for. I have tried to give you a starting point to help you navigate your way through the grocery store. You may find another brand or food item that better fits your needs.

One of the biggest changes that can positively enhance your physical health is to throw out the idea of what a breakfast typically looks like for you or your family. Is it possible to begin the day with foods that are not as acidic as typical breakfast foods tend to be? You can prepare a light lunch instead of the typical breakfast foods. Examples include soup, salad, cream of buckwheat, a smoothie, a wrap, gluten-free toast, rice, organic chicken nuggets with a veggie, etc.

The idea here is tri-fold:

1. Switching a food product from conventional to organic will reduce the amount of pesticides, GMO's, chemical fertilizers, preservatives, artificial colors, artificial flavors, fatty oils, possibly reduce added sugar and salt, and reduce other man-made chemicals. The idea is to get away from the mass marketed junk and processed foods and back to a more "clean" diet. For example, eating an organic pop-tart is better than a conventional pop-tart because you have eliminated most of the chemicals. However, it still may not provide the nutritional support your body requires (it is an acidic food). There is not a lot of nutritional value in any type of pop-tart. Yes, you have eliminated chemicals, but remember the importance of using foods to increase the state of alkalinity in your blood and decreasing foods that are acidic.

2. Reducing the amount of processed and packaged food you consume (whether it is organic or conventional) and increasing foods that provide the proper nutrients (fruits, vegetables, nuts, seeds, legumes, gluten free grains, etc.) is

something to consider. When you increase these nutrients, you will reduce the amount of packaged and processed foods that you purchase. You will also be reducing the acidic build-up in your body that can be attributed to these foods.

3. Is it possible to increase foods that are alkalizing (vegetables) and decrease foods that are acidic? For example, can you eat healthy for six days and on the seventh day enjoy your favorite meal, snack, beverage, or dessert? If you find that challenging, can you eat healthy for five days and enjoy your favorite foods for two days? The other thing to consider is can you eat a meal with foods that are eighty percent alkalizing (vegetables) and twenty percent acidic? If that is too much, can you try sixty percent alkalizing foods and forty percent acidic? Can you work your way up to the desired amount?

The items listed below can be found at your local grocery store, Whole Foods, Target, or your local health food store. These items should not replace a veggie loving diet. You can use them to help you transition to a more plant based diet. You can go to http://www.natural-health-zone.com for a list or chart of foods that are more alkalizing (maybe keep on refrigerator for meal planning purposes). Scroll down on the left hand side of the homepage and click on alkaline diet. The printable acid/alkaline food list is toward the bottom of the page. Another great resource is the book pH Miracle, by Robert O. Young. It is a great read and on pages 94-95 and 99 you will see the list of fruits and vegetables that are more or less acidic and alkalizing. Everyone can benefit from these lists. If you suffer from a digestive disorder, symptoms, or another illness, it might make sense to familiarize yourself with foods that decrease sugar and acidity and those that increase necessary nutrients. For example, a banana is considered acidic for someone trying to heal from Candida because of the sugar content even though it contains potassium, vitamin B, magnesium, vitamin C, and so on. A lemon is more alkalizing to the body and it contains less sugar. Can you incorporate more lemon in your daily diet and eat bananas in moderation? If you do not have any health issues, can you simply enjoy all fruits in moderation?

I want us all to enjoy a favorite dessert, a yummy meal, ice cream in the summer, candy on Halloween, cake at birthday celebrations, and a treat out at a sports game, concert, or movie. I am not suggesting to anyone that we should not enjoy these things every once in a while. I am suggesting our kids are on overload and it would be helpful to bring their food consumption back into balance. The food choices they make now and in the future will absolutely affect their overall health and well-being.

Instead of:	Choose:	Comment:	Common Product Brands:
Soda, juice boxes, lemonade, sweet teas, sports drinks, fruit juices, and frozen Juices	Water Kefir (probiotic) Zevia (soda) Green tea Organic juice boxes Coconut milk/ water	Your kitchen sink is probably not a clean water source.	Dasani – purified individual water bottles Gallon jugs of distilled water For reverse osmosis water systems visit (www.lowes.com) (www.zevia.com) (www.blueskysoda. com) (www.lifewaykefir.com) (www.scojuice, com) (www.rwknudsenfam-ily.com) Zero water filtration system (www.zerowa-ter.com)

Instead of:	Choose:	Comment:	Common Product Brands:
Yogurt and cheese	Organic yogurt and cheeses Daiya is a dairy, gluten, and soy free cheese alternative (www.daiyafoods.com) Go Veggie cheese is another dairy alternative (www.goveggiefoods.com) Dairy-free yogurt brands include: So Delicious (www.sodeliciousdairy-free.com) Almond Dream (www.almond-breeze.com)	A large number of cheeses contain an ingredient called rennet. Rennet is an enzyme from the lining of the stomach of a calf or other young animal. It is used in the cheese making process to help solidify the cheese.	Stony field Farm(www.stonyfield.com) Horizon (www.horizondairy.com) Organic Valley (www.organicvalley.coop) Stonyfield Farm yogurt tubes (www.stonyfield.com) Applegate Farm cheese (www.applegatefarms.com)
Popsicles/ice cream	Organic ice cream Almond milk ice cream Tofu ice cream sandwiches Frozen desserts that are dairy-free	You can try cold treats made from almond, coconut, or soy milk. Almond Dream (www.almond breeze.com) So Delicious (www. so deliciousdairyfree.com) Soy Dream (www.tastethe-dream.com)	Stonyfield Farm (www.stonyfield.com) Julie's organics (www.juliesorganic.com) Tofutti Brand (www.tofutti.com) Annie's (www.annies.com) Amy's (www.amys.com) Alden's (www.aldensi-cecream.com) Lifeway (www.lifeway.com)

Instead of:	Choose:	Comment:	Common Product Brands:
Frozen breakfast food including: waffles, pancakes, hash browns, breakfast sandwiches, bacon, sausages, and sugar cereals	Organic hash browns Oatmeal a piece of fruit smoothie healthy cereal trail mix raw vegetables bowl of brown rice organic or gluten-free pancake mix eggs uncured bacon salad sweet potato hash w/ veggies soup cream of buckwheat glass of green juice (homemade) The options are limitless. Be creative!	Eliminate all processed breakfast foods. Turkey bacon is not a good substitute for bacon.	Applegate Farms – bacon and sausage (www.applegatefarms.com) (can buy in bulk; large selection of frozen foods typical to the average American diet) Cereals: Cascadian Farms (www.cascadianfarm.com) Kashi (www.kashi.com) Nature's Path (www.naturespath.com) Ezekiel (www.foodforlife.com) Mother's (www.mothersnatural.com) Pancake & waffle mixes: Nature's Path (www.naturespath.com) Hodgson Mill (www.hodgsonmill.com) Frozen Waffles: Van's (www.vansfood.com) Nature's Path (www.naturespath.com

Instead of:	Choose:	Comment:	Common Product Brands:
Frozen dinner entrees, prepared meals, frozen vegetables in a sauce, frozen desserts, and frozen meat products	Prepare your meals fresh		Newman's Own pizzas Udi's (gluten-free products) (www.udisfood.com) Amy's (www.amys.com) Cascadian Farms organic French fries or tater tots Sweet potato fries and tater tots Cascadian Farms organic frozen vegetables (www.cascadianfarm.com) Bell and Evans Chicken nuggets (www.bellandevans.com) (also comes in gluten free version) Applegate Farm meats Ezekiel sprouted grains (www.foodforlife.com) Food for Life brown rice tortilla's (www.foodforlife.com)

Instead of:	Choose:	Comment:	Common Product Brands:
Vegetable oil, partially hydrogenated oils, margarine, butter, and saturated fats	Cold pressed olive oil grape seed oil (also comes in a spray to replace artificial butter sprays) safflower oil hemp oil flaxseed oil macadamia, sunflower, and sesame oils avocado oil red palm oil organic butter/ spreads		Earth Balance natural butter spread (www. earthbalancenatural. com) Oils: Newman's Own (www.newmansown. com) Spectrum Naturals (www. spectrumorganics.com) Woodstock foods (www. woodstock-foods.com)
Seasoned potato chips, cheese balls and curls, and tortilla chips (basically the entire chip aisle of the grocery store)	Plain chips (less ingredients) Veggie chips Pita chips Organic chips Sweet potato chips Pirate Booty Gluten-free chips Bean/flax chips		Pirate Booty (www. piratebrands.com) Nature for Life sprouted grain tortilla (I sprinkle with olive oil and fresh seasoning and bake in oven. Can be used as a chip or use as a replacement for taco shells. I break into pieces and make a taco salad. Can also be used as a chip.) Food Should Taste Good Natural Tortilla Chips (www.foodshould tastegood.com) RW Garcia chips (www. rwgarcia.com)

Instead of:	Choose:	Comment:	Common Product Brands:
Boxed oatmeal, pop-tarts, and breakfast bars	Organic steel-cut oats in bulk organic pop-tarts organic and/or gluten-free breakfast and granola bars		Nature's Path (www.naturespath.com) Annie's (www.annies.com) Health Valley (www.healthvalley.com) Cascadian Farms (www.cascadianfarm.com) Kashi (www.kashi.com) ClifKids (www.clifbar.com)
Soy sauce	Bragg Liquid Aminos (not fermented and Non-GMO) Tamari (fermented soy sauce)		Bragg Liquid Aminos (www.bragg.com)
Ketchup, mustard, mayonnaise, barbeque sauce, and pickle relish	Choose organic brands		Heinz (www.heinzfoodsservice.com) Spectrum (www.spectrumorganics.com) Annie's (www.annies.com)
Herbs	Replace bottled herbs with organic brands. Plant your own herbs outside in the summer or inside in the winter	You can plant basil, parsley, cilantro, mint, thyme, rosemary, or whatever you like.	Seedsofchange.com www.sustainable-seedco.com Simply Organic (www.simplyorganic.com) McCormick (www.mccormickgourmet.com)

Instead of:	Choose:	Comment:	Common Product Brands:
Enriched white pasta	You can chose a whole wheat pasta (contains gluten) an organic version of any type of pasta Ezekiel sprouted grain pasta Quinoa super grain pasta brown rice pasta	Our favorite gluten-free pasta is Bionature (www. bionature.com) Another yummy brand of pasta that is gluten free is made by Andean Dreams (www. andeandream. com)	(www.quinoa.net) (www.foodforlife.com) (www.ricepasta.com)
Enriched white flours including breads, pancake and waffle mixes, and cakes	spelt flour millet flour amaranth flour arrowroot flour buckwheat flour brown rice flour Look for organic boxed muffin and cake mixes. (these flours are gluten-free)		Flour: Bob's Red Mill (www. bobsredmill.com) Arrowhead Mills (arrowheadmills.com) Pancake mixes: Arrowhead Mills Nature's Path Red Mill

Instead of:	Choose:	Comment:	Common Product Brands:
Soups in cans and boxes	Make your own soups with organic beef, chicken, and vegetable stocks. Include organic vegetables and your new pasta.	Wolfgang Puck Health Valley Organic	Broths: Swanson (www. swanson. campbellskitchen.com) Pacific Natural Foods (www.pacificfoods. com) Soups: Wolfgang Puck (www. wolfgangpuck.com) Health Valley (www. healthvalley.com)
Salad dressings	Make your own using lemon, limes, herbs, and olive oil	There is the option of buying organic bottled dressings.	Seeds of Change (www. sustainable seedco.com) Annie's (www.annies. com) Newman's Own (www. newmansown.com) Organic Ville (organicvillefoods.com)
Deli meats and hot dogs	Choose deli meat that is nitrate-free and organic if possible.	Most Boar's Head deli meats are nitrate-free but not organic	Can order online as well at Applegate Farms (www.applegatefarms. com)

Instead of:	Choose:	Comment:	Common Product Brands:
Cookies	Organic brands or brands with fewer ingredients Gluten-free: Udi's (www.udisfood.com) Gluten-free cookies that you can bake and taste similar to nestle is made by a company called Immaculate (www.immaculatebaking.com) These are also dairy-free and nut-free.	Reduce intake of sugar products altogether.	Newman's Own (www.newmansownorganic.com) Late July (www.latejuly.com) BARBARA'S (www.BarbaraBakery.com) Country Choice Organics (www.countrychoiceorganics.com) Kashi (www.kashi.com) Immaculate Baking Co. (cookie dough) (www.immaculatebaking.com)

Instead of:	Choose:	Comment:	Common Product Brands:
Candy and gum	Organic or more natural products chocolates, lollipops, gum, candy, and mints	This is a tough thing to eliminate from a child's diet. Sugar-free candies are not a good substitute as they contain artificial ingredients and sweeteners. Can we reduce the amount of sugar our kids are consuming on a daily and weekly basis?	Gummy bears/worms/ jelly beans All Naturals (www. surfsweets.com) Chocolate bars and mints: Newman's Own Organics (www.newmansownor- ganic.com) Justin's (www.justins. com) Dagobah (www. dagobachocolate, com) Green and Blacks (www.green andblacks. com) Licorice – Panda (www.pandalicorce. com) Lollipops – Yummy Earth (www.yummyearth. com) Ricochet Sours (look and taste like Smarties candy) Emerald Forest (www. EmeraldForestSugar. com) Yummy Earth Organics (www.yummyearth. com) Glee Gum (www. gleegum.com)

Instead of:	Choose:	Comment:	Common Product Brands:
Canned vegetables	Choose fresh fruits and vegetables. It is my understanding that the cans are coated with chemicals to preserve products.		
Processed fruit strips, fruit pieces, fruit ropes, and fruit roll-ups	Chose organic or natural fruit strips and pieces. You eliminate most of the artificial ingredients.	Remember this item is high in sugar whether conventional or organic.	Annie's Organic fruit bunnies (www.annies.com) Clifkids twisted fruit (www.clifkid.com) Stretch Island fruit strips (www.stretchisland. com) Yummy Earth organics (www.yummyearth. com)
Artificial sweeteners		Avoid artificial sweeteners and refer to sugar for substitutes	
Applesauce	Organic		(www.santacruz.com) (www.vermontvillage-applesauce.com)
Boxed potatoes, macaroni and cheese, and rice	I have replaced with brown rice, quinoa, sweet potatoes, or basmati white rice. Both Annie's and Kraft carry a line of organic and chemically reduced products.	Add your own spices to rice and stay away from boxed rice.	You can find rice either in the organic section of your supermarket or in the bulk section. Kraft organic macaroni and cheese (www. kraftfoodsgroup.com) Annie's macaroni and cheese (www.annies. com) Simply Organic (www. simplyorganic.com)

Instead of:	Choose:	Comment:	Common Product Brands:
Sugar, High Fructose Corn Syrup	Organic white or powdered sugar pure cane sugar Xylitol Stevia brown rice syrup honey	Sugar should be eliminated from diet as much as possible, including the ones I just listed as an alternative. They are a better option though in moderation. All of the conversion rates for sugar that you need for baking purposes are labeled on the package or you can refer to websites as well.	Xylitol products: (www. emeraldforestxylitol. com) Stevia products: (www.stevia-products. com) (www.nunaturals.com) Brown rice syrup products: (www.lundberg.com) different types of organic sugars: Wholesome (www. OrganicSugars.biz) Woodstock (www. woodstock-foods.com)
Maple syrup	Agave nectar Organic blue agave Stevia powder Organic powdered sugar	Again, can you reduce sugar intake of any kind?	(www. madhavasweeteners. com) (www. wholesomesweetners. com) (www.naturals.com)

Instead of:	Choose:	Comment:	Common Product Brands:
Italian and plain breadcrumbs, seasoning packets including chili, fajita, Creole, and chipotle, and several options for batter mixes	Brown rice bread crumbs Organic seasoning packets	Most conventional seasonings include MSG, artificial flavorings and colors, and soy and gluten derivatives	Hol-grain (www.Hol-grain.com) Edward and Sons (www.edwards andson.com) McCormick spices (www.mccormick.com) Simply Organic seasoning packets (www.simplyorganic.com)
Salt	Himalayan salt Real Salt		Redmond real salt (www.realsalt.com)
All types of crackers	Healthier crackers that are organic or have fewer ingredients Gluten-free crackers Rice crackers	I would stay away from crackers that come in rainbow colors and have enriched flour.	Annie's – (www.annies.com) Kashi – (www.kashi.com) Late July – (www.latejuly.com) www.glutino.com bluediamond.com www.vansfoods.com
Baby food	Organic or make your own		

Instead of:	Choose:	Comment:	Common Product Brands:
Breads	Can you explore gluten-free breads?	reduce artificial colors, preservatives, HFCS, and enriched white flour	Udi's (www.udisfood.com) Rudi's (www.rudisbakery.com) Ezekiel bread (www.foodforlife.com) Deland Bakery (www.deland bakery.com) (organic and gluten free breads)
Eggs	Organic/cage free		Local farmer's market Organic Valley (www.organicvalley.com)
Tomato sauce	Organic		Muir Glen (www.muirglen.com) Amy's (www.amys.com) Organic Ville (www.organicvillefoods.com)
Nuts/seeds	Nuts: Almonds, walnuts, pine nuts, pecans, and brazil nuts. Seeds: sunflower, pumpkin, flax, chia, hemp, and sesame. Peanuts and cashews can be high in mold.	Nuts make a healthy snack and you can add seeds to anything. I would stay away from nuts found in the aisles of grocery store. Most have been freeze dried and processed. Can you try raw nuts and seeds? You can soak in water for a few minutes or overnight.	You can buy in the bulk section of the grocery store, Whole Foods, or Target.

Instead of:	Choose:	Comment:	Common Product Brands:
Peanut Butter (tends to be higher in mold than other nuts)	Organic	You can also try almond butter, hazelnut butter, sunflower seed butter, and tahini butter (sesame seed)	Smucker's (www.smuckers.com) Woodstock (www.woodstock-foods.com) Earth Balance (www.earthbalancenatural.com)

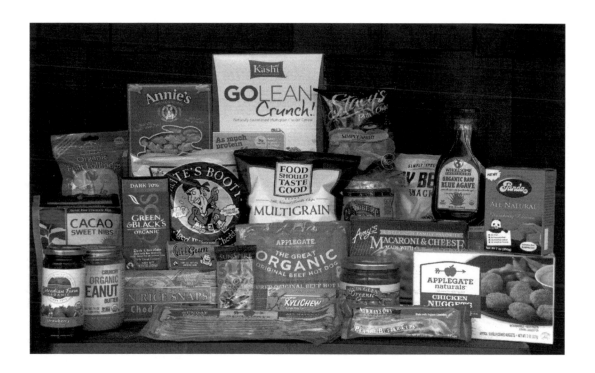

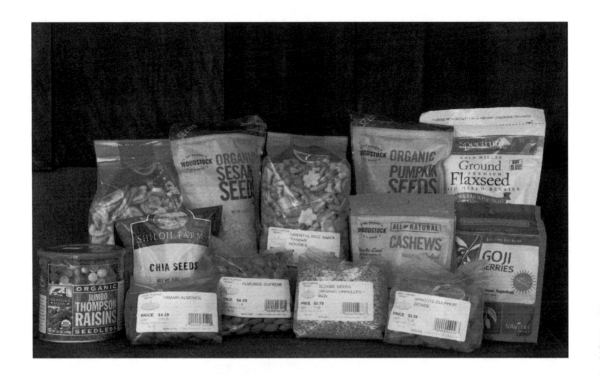

Other Food/Snack Ideas:

- Hummus with veggies
- Salsa/homemade guacamole
- smoothies
- Soups
- Wraps
- Salads
- Avocado with tomato or cucumber
- Flax chips
- Vegetables (raw, steamed, grilled, sautéed, and juiced) There are over hundreds of veggies to choose from.
- Homemade dressings
- Stuffed peppers or cabbage rolls
- Garlic and fresh herb gluten-free pasta
- Sweet potato mash/hash
- Homemade kale chips
- Baba ghanoush (eggplant dip with spices)

- Veggies, veggies, and more veggies!
- pizza's (gluten-free crust, organic cheese/Daiya cheese)
- Organic or gluten free mac and cheese
- Raisins and goji berries
- Sprouted grain or gluten-free pretzels
- Frozen fruit
- Rice cakes or crackers
- Sweet potato fries or taters
- Almond milk pudding
- Organic popcorn (the kind you make on the stove and not in the microwave)
- Celery with almond butter
- Homemade trail mix
- Again, more and more veggies!

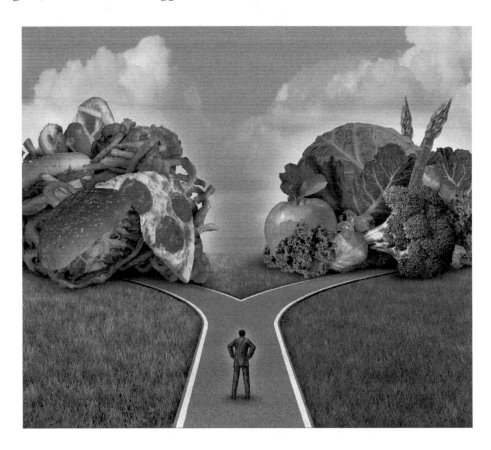

CHAPTER 15
My Turn

"When we are no longer able to change a situation, we are challenged to change ourselves."
~VIKTOR FRANKL

"For all your goodness I will keep on singing, 10,000 reasons for my heart to find."
— SONG, BLESS THE LORD OH MY SOUL

Everything I have learned, changed, and implemented in my house has been for the health and benefit of my children and family. By trying to help my son, I educated and shifted the way I think about food, taking care of myself, others, and the world we live in and share collectively. While this part of my journey as a parent was to help my son, many things have opened up to me on a personal level. This new awareness has inspired, taught, and is realigning the person I am today.

However, on November 5, 2012, my life came to a screeching halt. Or so I thought. I share my own personal medical journey with you now as it directly reflects the thoughts and ideas presented in this book. I believe my own medical journey presents a clear example of the possible coordination between modern medicine and the holistic approach to health. It also explores the entire holistic approach to health—body, mind, and spirit. I am a private person and am somewhat uncomfortable sharing my medical crisis with the world. However, I have chosen to share my story because I genuinely feel there is a larger message you can benefit from as it relates to your own health.

I have come to learn that good health does not have to be one way (modern medicine) or the other way (holistic). I believe we can use both to assist us in achieving quality health. Modern medicine and alternative health care practices can complement each other and be used together to promote healing when needed. I will say if you live your life with the intention of a holistic lifestyle, the need for conventional modern medicine will most likely diminish. I do believe both have helped contribute to the foundation of my successful surgery, recovery, and on-going post-surgery healing process.

October 31, 2012, started out as a typical day for me. I found myself out in nature enjoying a walk with our dog, Snickers.

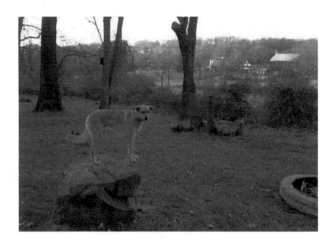

We were at our usual park that has provided both of us with many mornings of beauty and serenity. I was scheduled to have an MRI of the brain later in the day and it felt important to have the morning to clear my head and prepare myself for my appointment. I was reluctantly having the MRI as a precaution for some symptoms I had been experiencing for a few months. It was probably longer than a few months I was experiencing symptoms, but they were subtle. I did not pay much attention to them.

I had seen the registered nurse at my primary care doctor's office twice now for my on-going symptoms. I was being treated for a sinus infection and possible vertigo. I hesitantly took medication after a few months of no relief to see if it would help with my symptoms. The antibiotic and medication did not help with the symptoms and I found myself feeling progressively worse in a short amount of time.

The nurse practitioner noticed that something was not right with the movement of my right eye and referred me to an ENT specialist. I was experiencing no significant or new eye problems. Some of the symptoms I was experiencing were pressure headaches, minor balance issues, slight ringing in the ear with pressure, and numbness and tingling on the right side of my face. I was also beginning to lose the sense of taste on the right side of my mouth. Something was off and I couldn't quite put my finger on it. My walks with Snickers were getting shorter, it was becoming extremely disorienting to bend my head down in yoga class, and I had to stop playing tennis. I was noticing at the end of each day I was physically exhausted and would fall asleep in what felt like a matter of seconds. I wasn't ignoring the problem, but looking back I can admit I was not proactive about the situation either. I was engaging with the world and all that I was responsible for with the same speed and endurance as in the past.

One of the things I have learned recently is that it is important for me to learn to recognize and understand my body in a different way moving forward. Is there a forward? Shit, here come the negative thoughts about what could really be going on with me. What was my body trying to tell me? Was I listening and did I know how to listen? I had experienced symptoms that had progressively gotten worse or much more noticeable over the course of just a few months. The ENT specialist I was now seeing told me he wanted to rule out any problems associated with the brain. By having the anticipated negative MRI brain scan result, the doctor could eliminate the brain and focus on what I assumed was the problem, the inner ear.

How did I get to this point in my life? Should I be scared? This sounds serious now. At the time I was forty one year's young, in good health, and a somewhat healthy eater. Over the last few years I had slowly changed my diet from conventional foods to organic, swapped out typical cleaning supplies for less toxic versions, was beginning to simplify my life, and focusing more on what was important to me.

I was a witness to Frankie's incredible and life changing physical transformation and it would soon be my turn to learn more on the path to not only physical wellness, but spiritual and emotional wholeness as well.

On November 5, 2012, my husband and I walked into the doctor's office for the results of the MRI. I remember I kept telling Frank that he did not have to come with me. I felt that there was no need for him to miss half a day of work for this appointment. I could go to this consultation on my own and hear the negative test results by myself without intruding on his day. This was my first lesson. We all need support from our loved ones. I was glad he intuitively knew that this follow-up appointment was important to me, him, and our family.

As we arrived at the office, I made it a point to look into the nurse's eyes as she escorted us back to the examining room. I knew immediately that something was wrong. Shit again, what is wrong with me? Did I see pity, sorrow, or sadness staring back at me? No, it was more of a mother's love telling me everything was going to be OK. I also found it a bit unusual I had to go in to see the doctor and receive the anticipated negative results in person rather than receive the news over the phone.

I am confident that everyone has a day of reckoning or an experience of awakening. This was my moment. Life as I knew it would be forever changed in a matter of minutes. I did not understand how profound a thought and reality this was until a few months after surgery.

I was diagnosed with a large, benign brain tumor (Acoustic Neuroma or Vestibular Schwannoma). As you can imagine, I had a difficult time digesting and comprehending the words that were coming out of this doctor's mouth. The magnitude of the situation was terrifying! I know the doctor was having a difficult and sympathetic time delivering the news. I am grateful for his concern and expertise. As I sat listening to him, my first thought was that I was going to die. My second thought was how could I leave three young and beautiful children in this world without a mother? This seemed so unfair not to me, but to them. My third thought was how much I loved my husband and how upset I was that he was going to have to walk this journey with me, no matter the outcome? His life would be forever changed as well.

It took a few days for the shock and denial to diminish until I gathered my strength and courage to begin devising a plan of action. Where do I start?

An acoustic neuroma is a slow growing benign tumor. This type of tumor begins in the inner ear canal and as it grows it begins to push on the brain. There is no known medical cause for this type of tumor. According to the Acoustic Neuroma Association website, some studies have identified cell phone usage, defects in tumor suppressor genes, exposure to loud noises on a consistent basis, and prior exposure to head and neck radiation as potential causes. However, there is no specific and concrete medical answer. It just is. As my tumor grew it invaded the space between the ear and brain. That is the reason I was experiencing more and more symptoms. Because this type of tumor is slow growing, it is possible it has been with me for a few decades. It is incredible to imagine that through possibly part of my late teen years, college, marriage, traveling, sports, child bearing years, work, and life in general that I had "my silent friend" along for the ride.

I immediately began learning and educating myself about this type of tumor. Because the tumor was large in size and putting pressure on the brain stem, my options for medical treatment went down from three options to the one and only option that was medically viable for me, surgery. The only thing I knew was that I wanted it gone. The question for me now was how can I incorporate holistic approaches to the medical treatment plan now being laid out to me? Could I integrate both conventional medicine and a holistic approach to the successful removal and recovery from this tumor? How could I do that and where would I start?

As I contemplated my options, I wanted to find and consult with a doctor that would remove the entire tumor. This is a difficult procedure for many reasons. One of those reasons being that the cranial nerves are involved in this intricate surgery. The twelve cranial nerves in our brain enable many of our bodily functions including hearing, balance, taste, swallowing, facial movement, eye movement, coordination, and many more. Because the tumor was already large in size and given my physical symptoms, I knew from my research there were several cranial nerves already involved with this tumor. I was also frightened because the tumor was now pushing on the brain and putting pressure on the brain stem. I also knew in my heart that peeling the tumor off of these nerves would be difficult.

I obtained three recommendations for surgery from leading neurosurgeons. All agreed the tumor had to be removed. The next question for me was do I go with a surgeon who will remove most of the tumor, leaving a small section of it intact. This is done to minimize the disturbance to the nerves. Or do I go with the doctor who was extremely confident he could remove the entire tumor, leaving me with a 25 percent chance of complete facial paralysis on the right side. Leaving a small piece of the tumor intact has the potential to increase the chances of regrowth. I felt it was better emotionally to have the entire tumor removed. Was this doctor overly confident in his abilities to remove the entire tumor? What if he disturbed the nerves? What would the outcome be for me? Could I live with facial paralysis, headaches, swallowing problems, eye issues, facial drooping, or worse? How do I weigh all of these options while making the best decision with the best possible outcome for a full recovery for me?

I talked with my husband, family, friends, doctors, and alternative health care practitioners about my situation. I decided to schedule surgery for January 24, 2013, at one of the country's most premiere and leading hospitals on brain tumors. I chose the doctor who told me he was going in my brain to excise the entire tumor. After much thought, prayer, and reflection, I decided this was the best path for me. I was accepting of my choice and felt confident in my decisions thus far. I was scared and confused, but knew this was the right decision for me.

I contemplated why I had developed a brain tumor in the first place. How can I undergo such an invasive medical procedure and finish this book that focuses more on the importance of holistic principles? What is the higher message that now stares at me when I look in the mirror every morning? What was God's plan for me and did I have the faith to walk down this path with love and courage?

The thinking and reasoning behind why this was happening could be endless for me. I am a very concrete, visual, and critical thinker. There was definitely a lot of information that I could process at the time. I did not fail in this department and tried to process as much information about my type of brain tumor as I could ingest. Ultimately though, does any of this matter? Yes and no. Yes, it was my job to gather information about this type of tumor and the surgical approaches to removing it. I researched hospitals, neurosurgeons, potential treatment options, past surgical results, complications, insurance issues, and on and on.

On the other hand, there was a part of me that did not care about any of this. Here I was in the present moment with a large tumor in my head with no known medical cause. I had to learn quickly how to graciously accept where I was in life. I was getting ready to place my life in the hands of medical professionals whom I had only physically recently met. I soon realized that I was just along for the ride. If I kept my eyes open I had the opportunity to experience many gifts along the way.

I also decided during the waiting period between diagnosis and surgery I would continue to use holistic therapies to bring my physical, spiritual, and emotional bodies into balance. I had decided to use modern, conventional medicine to try and eradicate my body of this invader. I also decided to continue to use holistic practices to strengthen my body and mind for the long haul ahead. I was working very hard on all aspects of my being and, at times, felt a profound sense of balance and peace. Physically, I continued on my organic diet as best I could at the time and took vitamins and supplements specifically recommended for this part of my journey. I walked when I felt strong enough to, took baths, napped when I needed a break, laughed more than ever, and enjoyed my time with family and friends in a way that I did not fully appreciate in the past. It was the first time in my life that I felt a deep sense of gratitude, freedom, and humility for all that was within and around me. I also received acupuncture, continued a meditative yoga class with some physical modifications, received body work, worked with a therapist to help me process all of this, and most importantly, prayed to God for guidance, peace, and comfort daily. My outlook was strong and hopeful. Ultimately though, I was learning that I was not in control of this situation.

I identified my concerns about surgery (death, anesthesia, stroke, seizures, facial paralysis, and the absolute unknown of where I was heading). My life's path was forever changing. How could it not? Would this life path end at surgery or did I need to prepare myself for life after surgery? Death was a frightening thought to me at the time (it still is, but is evolving) and I did not spend much time weighing myself down in my perceived negativity. I tried to do just the opposite and engaged life in a way that I had not done in the past. Don't get me wrong, I certainly had my moments, but I was absolutely being guided to the gifts of life - rather than or more than - the ideas I had about death.

I have a strong network of friends, family, and community that were by my side every step of the way and beyond. With my eyes open I waited as patiently as I knew how for the two and a half months to pass before surgery. What did I see as I tried to wait patiently? I could never put into words the emotions and feelings that arose inside of me as I was the recipient of so much love. I was scared, confused, angry, and in some physical discomfort. Yet somehow, I found or touched on Grace. Humility, love, sympathy, empathy, joy, faith, gratitude, forgiveness, humor, and hope became my teachers. I experienced the complete unselfishness of others on a level that I can only describe as Holy. I saw what God sees in each and everyone one of us, Divine Perfection. The kindness, meals, prayers, and support I received were genuinely overwhelming and truly remarkable to witness. I will always carry that gratitude with me for the rest of my life (thank you—you know who you are! Too many people to name personally, but I hold a special place in my heart for all of you). It was the love from others (strangers included) that opened my heart a little further. It has forever changed the person I am today! There is no antibiotic or medication that can give you what I received while waiting for surgery. The only thing I had to do was be willing to open my eyes and heart.

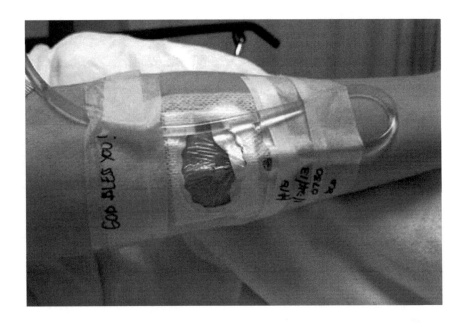

The day of surgery had arrived. Before going into the operating room one of the nurse's wrote this on my arm. It made me smile as I assumed she wrote, "God Bless You" on everyone's IV tape before being wheeled into surgery. One of the doctors who came to take me back to the operating room noticed it and asked me if I had written it. When I told him the nurse taking care of me had written it, he seemed quite surprised. He said something like, "Wow, she does not do that often." To me it was a sign that I was being cared for by higher powers that I am only beginning to understand.

The surgery lasted about seven hours. I will be forever grateful to the team of doctors and nurses who took such extraordinary care of me. The surgery was a success. The entire tumor was removed and I had come out on the other side. There were no immediate and physically dangerous complications as a result. I did, however, have many significant side effects including slight facial paralysis on the right side and extreme double vision. My right eye had lost the ability to move and focus. If you were standing in front of me, I saw you multiple times and from many different heights and angles. The team of doctors had to cut the vestibular/cochlear nerve during surgery. This left me permanently deaf in my right ear. That same nerve controls balance and I was now unsteady and wobbly. I also felt like I had just been run over by a highway full of semi-trucks.

I was expected to stay in the hospital for seven to ten days and was released after five. I was up walking (with assistance) around the hospital the next day and was weaned off medications permanently in a short amount of time. Modern medicine had done its job and I could not be more thankful. It was time to head home, hug my kids, and heal!

It has been approximately eighteen months since my surgery. The healing process has been a progressively slow transformation and a lesson on many things. Someone said to me that the healing process has its own agenda. It absolutely does and I am learning to move with it because it is always changing. My physical symptoms are getting better with time and assistance from medical and alternative practitioners. My side effects from surgery have evolved and I have physically overcome many obstacles on my path to the new me. I am learning to accept and overcome my new physical limitations. I look and act like I did before surgery, so it is difficult for people to understand the enormity of what I have been through and that I even have physical limitations. I think it was even hard for me to accept what had just happened to me.

However, my biggest and unforeseen obstacle in my healing process has been the anxiety (fear) that began about two months after surgery. I believe as I was processing the magnitude of all that I had just been through, the anxiety came out of nowhere and hit me like a ton of bricks. The anxiety was also probably due to all of the physical and sensory issues I was now facing and challenged with. Whatever the reason, this initial anxiety sent me straight down to the kitchen floor with my children looking on and back to the hospital by ambulance in a complete panic. This anxiety (it has gotten much better and I am fully confident I will get past this as well) is new to me. It is not easy for me to admit that my biggest struggle post-surgery is something that I created with my own thoughts. It is what it is. We all have struggles. This just happens to be one of many for me. I continue to work through this struggle today.

Not only was I slowly recovering physically from many side effects from surgery, I also now had to figure out how to navigate my way through the anxiety. It became very clear to me that the anxiety I now felt in every fiber of my physical being would be the most challenging part of this journey. The emotional and physical pain was excruciating. The fear I identified and worked through was that something post-surgical was going to happen to me. I was also afraid of all the sensory issues I was now experiencing. It was truly overwhelming and sent body into a panic. The question for me was do I now have the stamina to work through this new struggle and where do I start? How do I even begin to work on this issue when I am still trying to recover from brain surgery?

Initially, I asked my neurosurgeon for a prescription to help me lessen my body's response to the anxiety and fear. I felt like I needed something, anything to help. I was desperate and wanted out of this body that was causing so much unease. I wanted it to stop! How the *&%$% (use your imagination here) was I supposed to function and take care of three children with busy schedules?

My doctor told me he would not prescribe a medication for the anxiety. He continued by telling me I had to find a way to work through this issue on my own. My first thought was, "what"? Here I was struggling to overcome anxiety and to free my body from the physical results of stress and my out of control thoughts. I communicated my desire to have a medication (I do not like taking medications to begin with) to help me with this and he said, "No". Looking back it makes me laugh that I picked probably the only doctor in the country who would have said no in my circumstance. It took me about a week to realize what I needed to do for myself. This is, I believe, where the holistic approach to my life has supported me yet again. If I now had anxiety because of all of the new sensations on the side of my head where the tumor was removed, I had to figure out a way to overcome the anxiety. I did not know what the new me would be in the future or what that would look like physically. If these new sensations and sensory issues (continuous ringing with occasional crackling and zipping in the right ear, double vision and strain in the right eye, visual perception difficulties, numbness and tingling on the outside of my head at surgical sight, balance issues, single sided deafness that has created more challenges to me than I had anticipated, etc.) were here to stay, I knew I did not want to depend on a medication for the rest of my life. I did not want to become dependent on a daily pill to bring me peace of mind and to calm my body down. This would, without question, become the hardest thing I have ever overcome physically.

There is absolutely no judgment on anyone who takes an anti-anxiety pill to help with his or her pain or fear. We are all on different paths and this is mine. The feeling of anxiety is awful and truly indescribable. I can now empathize with anyone who suffers with this condition. The one thing I did do is go to my primary care doctor who gave me a prescription for Xanax. I keep a bottle in my purse in case I have a second panic attack or feel like I need it in certain situations or social environments (Yes, for those friends who are laughing about the purse, I do have one). I have yet to feel the need to open the bottle. I do have it just in case.

I knew all of the "alternative" practices that I have incorporated in my life before surgery would become extremely important in helping me overcome some of the gut wrenching anxiety I now felt. I immediately began to work with my therapist on this issue. I also began to receive acupuncture for stress relief, massage to relax my body, body work, and began taking yoga classes again. I began talking with God on a much deeper and more intimate level. I also started taking homeopathic remedies and recommended over-the-counter products to assist me in reducing anxiety and bringing my body back into balance. I developed a daily routine that was helping me get stronger physically and emotionally.

At about the same time that the anxiety began, I was referred to a nutritionist who was thought to be capable of helping me in not only reducing the anxiety, but assisting me with the entire healing journey. After speaking with her on the phone, she agreed to help me in a manner that would decrease all of my physical symptoms which ultimately would bring me some freedom and relief from the anxiety. I knew this would take time and that it would require commitment from me. I was ready to get started.

I have been working with the nutritionist for well over a year now. She is helping me better understand how proper nutrition can eliminate bodily inflammation, stress, and toxins, while at the same time promote health and vitality. The proper balance of nutritious, chemical free foods has the potential to accelerate any physical healing process including anxiety.

I am not sure if the proper balance of nutrition could have prevented my tumor from developing or growing in the first place. However, I am now using foods to strengthen my body and mind. I also believe I am providing my body with a fighting chance of not having to experience this tumor regenerating itself again. I have also come to believe and accept faithfully that most things happen in life for a divine reason and purpose. I don't always like it. However, I am learning to move with it, instead of against it.

Just as my physical and emotional needs have changed, so have the skills I have acquired to assist me on my journey. I would like to highlight some of the things I have done personally to assist me physically and emotionally. For anyone who is ready to make some changes, a good starting point is to locate and communicate with a homeopathic practitioner or nutritionist in your area. It is my hope I am able to reach the one person or maybe a few individuals' who find themselves in a difficult situation, don't know where to turn, want to try something different, and who resonate with the writing in this book.

I have taken a deeper look at my own diet. I continue to eliminate or diminish foods that no longer serve me. Now I am increasing foods that help the healing process and am providing my body with the proper nutrients (in much larger quantities) to sustain maximum health. I am decreasing foods that cause acidity and increasing foods that are alive, vibrant, and packed with nutritional goodness. This is a process that has been an on-going and ever changing learning curve for me that takes determination, commitment, a healthy attitude, and a deep sense of hope. It is also a practice that may need professional guidance.

I continue to utilize many of the recommendations I have highlighted throughout this book already. My eating habits have changed throughout the years as a direct result of Frankie's medical abyss, my own medical crisis, and the new information I am learning as it relates to food, our digestive systems, medicine, and our world. Below is a list of foods and things I have done in the last two years to assist in my recovery. I have increased, decreased, or eliminated these steps as my body and mind have become stronger and more in balance. While foods are an important part of healing and staying healthy, I also believe that taking care of ourselves emotionally and spiritually is just as important!

- Reduction or elimination of foods that cause inflammation in the body. For me that included soda, meat, chocolate, and some dairy. I try to eat consciously and make good decisions.

- Reduction of foods that contain soy, gluten, and corn (This includes most packaged, processed, and fast foods.).

- Implementation of daily vitamin protocol that helped to strengthen my body and nourish my brain. Some of these vitamins include vitamins B and C, Omega 3, calcium, and probiotics.

- Proper hydration. An increase in pure and clean water as well as an increase in liquid intake to also include: vegetable broth, juicing, and a morning smoothie.

- Incorporation of nuts and seeds into daily eating habits (almonds, pecans, walnuts, and flax, chia, hemp, pumpkin, and sunflowers seeds).

- An increase in the amount of beans consumed.

- An increase in more diverse vegetables and in much larger quantities (steamed, sautéed, broiled, juiced, and eaten raw). Some of these vegetables include: spinach, broccoli and cauliflower, onion, garlic, peppers, spaghetti and butternut squash, kale, asparagus, Brussels sprouts, peas, green beans, eggplant, Swiss chard, radishes, cabbage, cucumber, sprouts, sweet potatoes, carrots, celery, Bok Choy, fresh herbs, and different types of lettuce to name a few.

- An increase in fruits including: lemons, limes, grapefruit, avocados, raw tomatoes, and green apples. I also now eat blueberries, blackberries, kiwi, mango, bananas, pineapple, clementines, and strawberries in moderation due to the higher sugar content.

- A switch in my family's bread source. There is a bakery in Florida (www.delandbakery.com) that provides products that significantly reduce the ingredient list, are gluten-free, organic, and have a higher nutritional value.

- Utilization of homeopathic remedies to assist with the surgical wound site and feelings of anxiety.

- Use of other homeopathic remedy products to help with the anxiety. Natural Calm is a powder magnesium supplement (www.naturalvitality.com) and Rescue Remedy (www.bachflower.com) provides natural stress relief. It comes in a spray, gum, drops, and chews. There are also flower essences made by the same company that can be added to a liquid to help with specific emotional concerns.

- Warm salt and aromatherapy baths

- Castor oil packs (www.edgarcasey.org). Castor oil has been used since ancient times to treat many conditions. It increases circulation, detoxes the body, provides support to lymphatic system, and can act as a laxative.

- I also began to talk to myself differently through positive affirmations and accepting myself (all of me) on a deeper level (This takes practice and an open mind. It is still a work in progress and sounds funny to me just writing it out on paper). When you go through a life altering surgery you tend to view the world differently. At least I do. I have found ways to reduce my daily activity and carve out more time for me. I am learning how to take care of myself on a much deeper and consistent basis. I am focusing more on what is important to me (family, friends, this project, learning to slow down, saying no on occasion when asked to volunteer my time, taking care of myself, learning to just "be", having fun, and most importantly, growing spiritually).

- I use audiobooks and attend workshops that provide tools, resources, information, and a positive outlook to assist in my approach to life and the anxiety. I try never to be critical of myself for having anxiety in the first place. I have developed strategies and techniques to help should I begin to feel anxious.

- I use nature and listening to music as a way to bring calm into my daily routine. I have been back to my morning walks with Snickers for a while now!

- As I stated previously, I used therapy to help me process this life change and transition. I also continue with massage, yoga, meditation, acupuncture, nutrition counseling, and bodywork (Reiki).

- I have begun to eliminate or at least to become aware of daily stressors and how I can utilize my knowledge to reduce them.

- I now get the proper amount of sleep most nights and enjoy a nap on occasion.

My anxiety has diminished significantly and my physical symptoms are getting better as a result of time and taking care of myself. As I learn how to navigate my way around my physical limitations, I feel blessed for many reasons. One of those reasons is for having had to travel down this road. It has forever changed the course of my life. Yes, there is a part of me that is grateful for this life experience. It has been a long, difficult, scary, frustrating, and challenging process. It has also been a profound journey on hope and love. It has changed my entire life and the way I think about life. I will forever be grateful because it has taught me and is teaching me many valuable lessons about life, who I am, and where I am going.

I do not have charts, graphs, statistics, or scientific data to quantify the effects of holistic health on my successful surgery and healing process. I will leave that to others to judge and evaluate. Modern medicine did its job from beginning to end. I put my faith and life in a team of doctors that are very scientifically educated and skilled. Thank you to Dr. Tamargo, Dr. Chien, and the entire team at Johns Hopkins Hospital for taking such extraordinary care of me.

Words could never express my gratitude to you, Frank, for taking such good care of me in the hospital and at home. You gave me the time to heal and it was a gift beyond measure! You allowed me the opportunity to focus on myself which was so important in this journey. You became Mr. Mom and selflessly took on more responsibility than one person should have to carry. I LOVE YOU!

I also put my trust and faith in a group of holistic practitioners who have slowly over time helped me on many, many different levels. Gratitude and love to Jenny, Dawn, Lydia, Julie, Dr. B, and Christine - my angels on earth.

Thank you Mom and Dad for your unconditional love and support during this difficult time and always.

I also believe that God and His mighty choir of angels have been with me every step of the way. A friend told me before surgery that I was going to have an incredible God story to tell. She could not have been more right.

This journey opened my eyes to what I have been searching for most of my adult life which is a deep, intimate, and faith filled relationship with God. Mine is a quiet, sometimes questioning, and an increasingly confident journey to know and accept God in all ways and at all times.

However I chose to look at this journey and however you choose to interpret my experience, the holistic ideas that I hold close are helping to empower me to become the person I was always meant to be. It is my hope as you evolve as a human being that you are open to the idea of change and looking at your health from a different perspective. I happened to begin doing that by changing my thought process about disease and food as it relates to my son's health and now my own health. Frankie laid the foundation and opened the door for me to begin looking at foods as a way to accelerate healing. I have realized that much of the physical suffering we all experience can be diminished, sometimes completely alleviated, and most certainly controlled by choosing to let go of the "modern" manner in which we eat and choose to take care of ourselves. I am not the "poster child" for living a healthy life. Actually, it is just the opposite. My past is anything but ideal. I have grown in the last few years and am doing my best to make good choices, as I know we all are! I am learning to better support myself physically and emotionally.

One thing I do know is that we would all benefit from simplifying our lives. We are losing control of our lives (I was) and what is truly important to each one of us. I was a typical, over worked mother who always put herself last. Through the years we have created stress on a monumental level. This stress is not good for us and it is not good for our children. Is it possible to teach ourselves and our children how to simply slow down and enjoy? If you ask me this should be a class taught in every elementary, middle, and high school across the country along with proper nutrition, understanding your body, meditation, and, dare I say it, spirituality. Oops. I said it.

I have no idea why I began this writing project and can't believe that I am almost done. I am not sure where the words came from or how it all came together. I know I did not embark on this project for me. As I have grown over the last few years, I have come to appreciate all of the universal forces that bring a project to fruition.

It is my hope this book has touched you on some level and that you are open to considering looking at your health and the health of your family from a new perspective. I implore you not to wait until a health crisis to consider making some necessary changes to the *toxic* world we are living in today. We can no longer sit by and idly watch what is happening in our society. We must find our voice individually and collectively. There is too much at stake beginning with your family's health.

I am much more aware of the life changing medical conditions that are affecting my generation of men and women. The stories I am hearing are sad, scary, and in all of our communities. I have heard stories of individuals in their thirties and forties recently that have been diagnosed with or have died as a result of breast cancer, depression, blood cancers, anxiety, asthma, irritable bowel syndrome, leaky gut syndrome, colitis, other major digestive disorders, allergies, MS, high blood pressure, brain tumors (more than I ever imagined), fibromyalgia, high cholesterol, pneumonia, chronic and unexplained symptoms, stroke, infertility, heart attack, skin conditions, brain cancer, other cardiovascular diseases, sudden death, and many more. These stories concern me for several reasons. I would have thought it would be our parent's generation (the baby boomers) who would be experiencing most of these diagnoses, not mine. I do not say that with a conceited "it-can't-happen-to-me" attitude because I know it can, but more as a connection to the natural progression of getting older. Nor do I wish these conditions on anyone. I do, however, believe that something is fundamentally wrong with our current daily environment.

I firmly believe the toxins we are unknowingly exposed to on a daily basis are unequivocally accelerating disease, symptoms, and illnesses. The chemicals that we are exposed to on a daily and continuous basis are creating chaos for our bodies. If it is true (depending on who you ask or how you choose to look at chemicals in our environment today) that chemicals and toxins are contributing to illness and disease on a level we are now only beginning to experience, study, and accept, I have one final question remaining for you to ponder and explore. What will the state of our children's overall health be in the future if disease is accelerating at a faster rate now than in the past and chemicals are being created, manipulated, and introduced over and over again into every single facet of their daily lives? Think about the children you know. How many of them are facing health issues, diseases, chronic symptoms, or behavioral concerns? No one truly knows the short and long term negative consequences to their bodies and cognitive functioning as a result of their toxic environment. Are we truly OK with accepting that answer? Are we willing to simply pass on these gigantic problems to our children?

I believe our children are the last stand we have as a collective unit to bring back into balance the issues that are hurting us today. If our kids are not educated or even introduced to these issues, they cannot pass this important information onto their children. Future generations will be more stressed out (is that even possible?), less able to cope with these stressors, more sick, more "busy", taking more medications, dying younger, suffering more, and will not have the tools to live a more natural or holistic lifespan. Not only will there physical bodies be out of balance, but their emotional and spiritual bodies will be as well. This is why I have taken the time to write this book!

We cannot stop the dying process, but we can educate ourselves on how to travel down our own unique life path with the necessary wisdom needed to maintain or enhance each of our physical journeys. We have the opportunity to enhance the quality of the remaining time we have been given on earth. I am not suggesting that tomorrow everybody needs to throw out everything in their kitchen and start over. Nor I am asking you to live your life the way that I do mine. I am, however, asking you to consider looking at the issues that I have laid out in this book with an open mind and with deep questioning. What is happening in our society and to our families affects us all! Living in today's world has many challenges. It is also a beautiful and mysterious gift! Educating ourselves on how to use the earth God has given us to create a safe and healthy environment is a responsibility we all share together. Whether we want to recognize, accept, and begin the necessary process of change or not is for you to decide. Be well!

CHAPTER 16
Resources for Families

"The ultimate test of a person's conscience may be his or her willingness to sacrifice something today for the future generations whose words of thanks will not be heard."

—GAYLORD NELSON

This chapter highlights some additional resources I have found over the last few years. These resources are full of information on a host of topics that relate to physical and emotional health, digestive health, food, and food education. These resources also explore what parents and individuals can do to create an environment that is healthy for you, your family, community, and all of us.

Please remember that throughout this book there are resources for you to consider as well. There is much to learn and share with others. I hope you take the time to do some reading and researching for yourself.

Topic: Candida and Digestive Health (most books also share information about nutrition, recipes, and food):

Candida by Jo Dunbar

Digestive Wellness by Elizabeth Lipski, Ph.D., CCN

The Candida Cure: Yeast, Fungus and Your Health by Ann Boroch, CNC

The PH Miracle by Robert O. Young and Shelley Redford Young

The Candida-Yeast Syndrome by Ray C. Wunderlich, Jr., M.D.

The Yeast Connection Handbook by William G. Crook, M.D.

Complete Candida Yeast Guidebook by Jeanne Marie Martin

How to Cope Successfully with Candida by Jo Dunbar

Digestive Wellness for Children by Elizabeth Lipski

You tube video on pH Miracle: www.youtube.com/watch?v=DdjLHIItiUE

www.nationalcandidacenter.com

www.annboroch.com

www.candidasupport.org

www.theyeastdiet.com

www.candidaresources.com

Topic: Food

Superfoods by David Wolfe

The Unhealthy Truth by Robyn O'Brien

Chew on This by Eric Schlosser & Charles Wilson

The Food Revolution by John Robbins

Gluten-free Diet by Shelly Case

The Real Food Revolution by Tim Ryan

Juicing, Fasting, and Detoxing for Life by Cherie Calbom

<u>Fat Chance: Beating the Odds Against Sugar, Processed Foods, Obesity and Disease</u>
by Robert Lustig

<u>The Food Babe Way</u> by Vani Hari

<u>Eat To Live </u>by Joel Fuhrman MD

www.sunfood.com

www.foodmyths.org

www.sweetsurprise.com

www.davidwolfe.com

www.livelovefruit.com

www.kriscarr.com

www.foodbabe.com

www.momsacrossamerica.com

Topic: Renewal and Awakening

<u>The Power is Within You</u> by Louise L. Hay

<u>You Can Heal Your Life</u> by Louise L. Hay

<u>Honor Yourself</u> by Patricia Spadaro

<u>Why People Don't Heal and How They Can</u> by Caroline Myss

<u>Dying To Be Me</u> by Anita Moorjani

Movie: The Secret

Topic: Chemical Fertilizers/Toxicity

<u>Fateful Harvest</u> by Duff Wilson

<u>Staying Healthy in a Toxic World</u> by Eugene A. Bolognese, DC

<u>Healthy Child Healthy World</u> by Christopher Gavigan

Movies: Food (You can rent some of these documentaries on iTunes, watch on Netflix or buy from Amazon.com):

Food, Inc.

The Future of Food

Our Daily Bread

Bad Seed: The Truth about Our Food

Dying to Have Known

Food Matters

King Corn: You Are What You Eat

Fowl Play: The Untold Story behind Your Breakfast

Fast Food Nation

Supersize Me

The Gerson Miracle

Vegucated

Forks over Knives

Fat, Sick & Nearly Dead

Fat, Sick & Nearly Dead 2

Hungry for Change

Killer at Large

Beautiful Truth

Defying Disease-Ted Talks

GMO OMG

Farmageddon

Vanishing Bees

Topic: informational Websites/Organizations

www.rodaleinstitute.org

www.soundstrue.com

www.gerson.org

www.youtube.com (enter your search question)

www.greenmedinfo.com

www.eomega.org

www.nrdc.org

www.bodymindinstitute.com

www.mindvalley.com

www.cornucopia.org

www.huffingtonpost.com

www.ewg.org

www.naturalnews.com

www.sustainabletable.org

www.mercola.com

www.kriscarr.com

www.foodbabe.com

www.cspinet.org

www.hippocratesinst.org

www.nutritionaction.com

Cookbooks:

The Amazing Acid Alkaline Cookbook by Bonnie Ross

100 Days of Real Food by Lisa Leake

The Eat-Clean Diet Cookbook by Tosca Reno

Crazy Sexy kitchen by Kris Carr

Eating the Alkaline Way by Natasha Corrett and Vicki Edgson

Topic: Vaccination and childhood diseases

Government resources:

www.cdc.gov/vaccines/vac-gen/additives.htm

CDC – information Contact Center #1-800-232-4636

www.cdc.gov/vaccines

To report a health problem that followed vaccination call the Vaccine Adverse Event Reporting System (VAERS) 1-800-822-7967

Public tracking/listing of adverse reactions to vaccines http://vaers.hhs.gov/data/data

CDC's Vaccines & Immunizations website -www.cdc.gov/vaccines

The National Vaccine Information Center - www.nvic.org

Resources that highlight concerns regarding vaccinations:

<u>Callous Disregard</u> by Dr. Andrew Wakefield

<u>Healing and Preventing Autism</u> by Jenny McCarthy and Jerry Kartzinel, M.D.

<u>The Vaccine Book</u> by Robert W. Sears, M.D., F.A.A.P.

<u>Evidence of Harm</u> by David Kirby

<u>The Nontoxic Baby</u> by Natural Choice

<u>Immunizations: The Reality Behind the Myth</u> by James Walene

www.youtube.com/watch?v=Xwfnd_WRkiU

www.immunize.org/concerns

www.callousdisregard.com

Topic: Therapy

www.holisticnetworker.com

www.byregion.net

www.naturalpsychotherapy.com

Topic: Holistic and naturopathic practitioners in your area

American Holistic Medical Association (AHMA)

http://www.holisticmedicine.org

National Center for Complementary and Alternative Medicine (NCCAM)

http://nccam.nih.gov/health/practitioner/index.htm

American Holistic Health Association (AHHA)

http://www.ahha.org

American Association of Naturopathic Physicians (AANP)

http://www.healthy.net/asp/Associations/aanp.asp

National Center for Homeopathy (NCH)

http://wwwhomeopathic.org

Topic: Nutritionists in your area

National Association of Nutrition Professionals (NANP) www.nanp.org

American Holistic Medical Association (AHMA) www.holisticmedicine.org

<u>Healthy Journeys: A Comprehensive Guide to Health Food Stores in the United States</u>

by Lance Norman and Heather Houk

You can contact me to discuss any questions you have or to schedule a consultation by phone. I can be reached at findingtheway2014@gmail.com

You can also follow me on twitter @findingtheway14 and Facebook @FindingtheWay

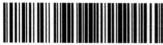

Made in the USA
Middletown, DE
14 May 2015